Feeding Cities

There is enormous current interest in urban food systems, with a wide array of policies and initiatives intended to increase food security, decrease ecological impacts, and improve public health. This volume is a cross-disciplinary and applied approach to urban food system sustainability, health, and equity.

The contributions are from researchers working on social, economic, political, and ethical issues associated with food systems. Its focus is on the analysis of and lessons obtained from specific experiences relevant to local food systems, such as tapping urban farmers' markets to address issues of food access and public health, and use of zoning to restrict the density of fast food restaurants with the aim of reducing obesity rates. Other topics considered include building a local food business to address the twin problems of economic and nutritional distress, developing ways to reduce food waste and improve food access in poor urban neighborhoods, and asking whether the many and diverse hopes for urban agriculture are justified.

The chapters show that it is critical to conduct research on existing efforts to determine what works and to develop best practices in pursuit of sustainable and socially just urban food systems. The main examples discussed are from the United States, but the issues are applicable internationally.

Christopher Bosso is Professor of Public Policy and Urban Affairs and Coordinator of the Consortium for Food Systems Sustainability, Health, and Equity at Northeastern University, Boston, USA. His areas of interest include food and environmental policy, science and technology policy, and the governance of emerging technologies.

Feeding Cities

Improving local food access, security, and resilience

Edited by Christopher Bosso

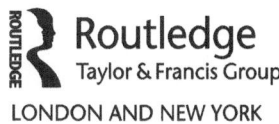

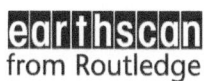

LONDON AND NEW YORK

First published 2017 by Routledge

2 Park Square, Milton Park, Abingdon, Oxfordshire OX14 4RN
711 Third Avenue, New York, NY 10017

Routledge is an imprint of the Taylor & Francis Group, an informa business

First issued in paperback 2018

British Library Cataloguing-in-Publication Data
A catalogue record for this book is available from the British Library

Library of Congress Cataloging in Publication Data
Names: Bosso, Christopher J. (Christopher John), 1956- editor.
Title: Feeding cities : improving local food access, security and sovereignty / edited by Christopher Bosso.
Description: London ; New York : Routledge, 2017. | Series: Routledge studies in food, society and environment | Includes bibliographical references and index.
Identifiers: LCCN 2016021374| ISBN 9781138647251 (hbk) | ISBN 9781315627137 (ebk)
Subjects: LCSH: Food supply--United States. | Food security--United States. | Sustainable agriculture--United States. | Urban agriculture--United States. | Public health--United States.
Classification: LCC HD9005 .F44 2017 | DDC 338.1/973--dc23
LC record available at https://lccn.loc.gov/2016021374

ISBN: 978-1-138-64725-1 (hbk)
ISBN: 978-0-367-02980-7 (pbk)

Typeset in Times
by Saxon Graphics Ltd, Derby

Contents

Figures

Tables

Contributors

Karen Banks is a senior program officer at the Johns Hopkins Center for a Livable Future, Johns Hopkins University, Baltimore, Maryland. She completed this review when she was a program manager at Share Our Strength, Washington, DC.

Janaki Blum is a master's degree candidate in the Department of Urban and Environmental Policy and Planning at Tufts University, Medford, Massachusetts.

Christopher Bosso is Professor of Public Policy and Urban Affairs at Northeastern University, Boston, Massachusetts.

Ashley Chaifetz is a social science research analyst in the Office of Policy Support at the USDA Food and Nutrition Service. She completed this research when she was a research associate at North Carolina State University, Raleigh, North Carolina.

Benjamin Chapman is an associate professor and food safety extension specialist in the department of Youth, Family, and Community Sciences at North Carolina State University, Raleigh, North Carolina.

Cara Cuite is an associate research professor in the Department of Human Ecology at Rutgers University, New Brunswick, New Jersey.

Sarita Daftary-Steel is Program Director for the Green Light District and the Williamsburg Leadership Center at El Puente (Brooklyn, NY), Project Consultant to Food Dignity, and former Project Director, East New York Farms! United Community Centers.

Jonathan Deutsch is Professor of Culinary Arts and Food Science at Drexel University, Philadelphia, PA.

Hedley Freake is Professor of Nutritional Sciences at the University of Connecticut, Storrs, Connecticut.

Suzanne Gervais is a senior extension associate in the Division of Nutritional Sciences, Cornell University, Ithaca, New York.

Phoebe Godfrey is Assistant Professor of Sociology at the University of Connecticut, Storrs, Connecticut.

Mehreen Ismail is a doctoral student at the Friedman School of Nutrition Science and Policy, Tufts University, Boston, Massachusetts.

Solomon H. Katz is Director of the Krogman Center for Research in Child Growth and Development, University of Pennsylvania, and CEO of the World Food Forum, Philadelphia, Pennsylvania.

Joseph Llobrera is a senior technical specialist at Insight Policy Research, Arlington, Virginia.

Chris Mancini is the Executive Director of Groundwork Somerville, Somerville, Massachusetts.

Daryl Marshall is former East New York Farms! Community Organizer and Youth Worker, United Community Centers.

Bakeyah Nelson is a public health consultant for Community Health Collaborative Consulting and a Generations Faculty Fellow for the Center for Generational Studies at the University of South Alabama, Mobile, Alabama. She completed this review when she was an assistant professor at the University of Houston, Clear Lake.

Austin Nijhuis is a senior research analyst with the Initiative for a Competitive Inner City, Boston, Massachusetts.

Thomas H. O'Donnell is Sustainability Coordinator at the U. S. Environmental Protection Agency, N.A.H.E., Region 3, Philadelphia, Pennsylvania.

Luisa Oliveira is a senior planner in the Mayor's Office of Strategic Planning and Community Development, City of Somerville, Massachusetts.

Christine M. Porter is an assistant professor and Wyoming Excellence Chair in Community and Public Health in the Division of Kinesiology and Health, University of Wyoming, Laramie, Wyoming.

Sandra Raponi is an associate professor of Philosophy at Merrimack College, North Andover, Massachusetts.

Lisa Robinson is the Director of Shape Up Somerville, a program of the Department of Health and Human Services, City of Somerville Massachusetts.

Erica Satin-Hernandez is the Coordinator of Shape Up Somerville, a program of the Department of Health and Human Services, City of Somerville Massachusetts.

Sara Shostak is Associate Professor of Sociology and Chair of the Health, Science, Society, and Policy Program at Brandeis University, Waltham, Massachusetts.

Michele Ver Ploeg is an economist with the Economic Research Service, U.S. Department of Agriculture, Washington, D.C.

David Vigil is Project Director for East New York Farms! United Community Centers.

Parke Wilde is Associate Professor at the Friedman School of Nutrition Science and Policy, Tufts University, Boston, Massachusetts.

Cathy Yungmann is Associate Professor of Communications, Cabrini College, Radnor, Pennsylvania.

Alexandra Zeitz is Manager of the Drexel Food Lab, Center for Hospitality and Sports Management, Drexel University, Philadelphia, Pennsylvania.

Kimberly Zeuli is Senior Vice President and Director of Research at the Initiative for a Competitive Inner City, Boston, Massachusetts.

1 What you want, when you want it?

Christopher Bosso

In March 2001 I travelled to Ames, Iowa to talk about the views held by environmental and animal welfare activists as part of a then-annual agricultural forum convened by the Center for Agricultural and Rural Development (CARD) at Iowa State University, one of the nation's great land-grant universities. Upon being invited to participate, I did what any good guest should do: I checked out my hosts. After all, I live in an East Coast city, teach at a large urban university, and have no experience whatsoever with "real" farming, so I wanted to understand what I was getting myself into. Equally important, I wanted to avoid embarrassing myself before the several hundred in attendance, including agricultural researchers, food industry officials, students, and, yes, a lot of Iowa farmers with time on their hands before spring planting. So I checked out the ISU College of Agriculture website to get a sense as to what it does.

The first image I came upon was not a farm, or pigs, or even that famous Grant Wood portrayal of the iconic American farm family. Instead I was presented with the image of a scientist in a white lab coat standing in front of a somewhat impressive-looking electronic analyzer of some sort. To be fair about it, subsequent visits to the College's website indicated that this image was but one of many faces of agriculture presented by the College – yes, I found barns and pigs – but that first image left an impression.

Here is why. The intended message of that image was, I suppose, "better farming, and better food products, through science." Fair enough. However, the image of the scientist in the white coat also inadvertently captured a critical issue at the heart of the Forum, whose theme that year was *Extreme Demands – Extraordinary Products*: the gap between the realities of agriculture as an industry and the attitudes Americans held in 2001 about personal health and their environment, about corporations, and, finally, about the role of the citizen in democratic decision-making.

The average American consumer, I observed to my audience, may not understand much about agriculture, but certainly had opinions on *food*, particularly its cost, quality, and safety. But an increasing number of Americans were becoming concerned about what they perceived as a food production system that had become concentrated in fewer and larger corporate hands, overly focused on maximizing production at the expense of the environment and animal welfare, and, in the wake of scares about Mad Cow disease and salmonella in chickens, seemingly more concerned with the economic interests of producers than the health and safety needs of the citizen-consumer. Americans may accept big companies like Cargill and Tyson for the goods and services they provide, but they nonetheless fear the distorting impacts of corporate power. In particular, while they want inexpensive and convenient food, they have doubts as to the degree to which producers will safeguard food safety. That 86 percent of Americans in one 2000 Harris Poll wanted mandatory labeling on products containing genetically modified organisms (GMOs) was an indication that the public had grown uneasy about the marriage of science and food.

In short, I said, Americans want someone to keep an eye on corporate America, to maintain a dynamic tension between the forces of the market and the forces of government. Groups that focus on consumer health, animal welfare, worker safety, and food purity are in a long tradition of American activism aimed at maintaining this balance. The good news, I concluded, was that Americans increasingly care about the conditions under which their food is produced. The *bad* news, for many in the audience, was that Americans increasingly cared about the conditions under which their food is produced.

Of course, such concerns have only become more acute since that March 2001 forum. The number, range, and size of advocacy groups focused any number of food-related issues has exploded. Food studies programs, once the near exclusive purview of agricultural schools like ISU, now proliferate in urban universities like my own, with new generations of students determined to fix the many ills they perceive about the dominant food system, if not the larger socioeconomic system of which it is part. The sheer volume of books and films critiquing some dimension of the food system now overwhelms us. Walmart, not Whole Foods, is the nation's largest retailer of organic fruits and vegetables. More Americans of many more types now care what is in their food and where it comes from, and demand all kinds of information, whether it contains GM variants, the country of origin, or whether it was fairly traded, humanely raised, or sustainably grown – whatever those terms might mean.

Those of us in urban America – which, if you include larger metropolitan areas, means most of us – flock to an ever growing number of farmers' markets and farm-to-table restaurants, commit to buying Community Supported Agriculture (CSA) shares, agitate to address urban "food deserts" and advocate for urban agriculture. We even care what is in the Farm Bill, that sprawling federal legislation that because of advocacy by consumer, environmental, and nutrition groups now includes at least some support for organic agriculture and "specialty" crops like fruits and vegetables, offers incentives for more ecologically sustainable production practices, and promotes healthier eating, even if it also continues to define, if not prop up, a dominant food system about which so many of us find fault.

In this regard, *it bears reminding*: Americans are accustomed to plentiful, diverse, convenient, and inexpensive food. To put it plainly, for *most* Americans the food system gives us what we want, when we want it, and at a price we're willing to pay. On average, we spend around 10 percent of net income on food, whether eaten at home *or* outside of it, the lowest level per capita in the world.[1] In human history terms, this is no small achievement. While the United States started out with advantages in arable land, water, and favorable growing conditions, today's abundance is also due to key characteristics of the food system as it evolved since the middle of the twentieth century. It is a food system that in many respects is an apt reflection of the norms of industrial efficiency: large scale, specialized, mechanized, technologically sophisticated, global in reach. If you live in Boston and want fresh blueberries in February, you can get them, shipped in by air from Chile. And it is all done by a relatively small group of producers. In 1940, nearly 31 million Americans, 25 percent of the population, worked the farm. In 2012 it was 3.1 million – a farming 1 percent feeding everyone else.[2]

And yet, as we know, that food system doesn't necessarily work for everyone, and its pathologies affect us all. Many (but certainly not most) of us worry that the dominant food system, while efficient, is too distant, unaccountable, and not sustainable. We worry that it emphasizes the production of inexpensive but unhealthy processed foods over healthier but (at the moment) more expensive fresh fruits and vegetables, or that the "cheap meat" model is ecologically harmful and ethically suspect. In some ways, we have the luxury of the affluent, worrying that the food system that gives most of us inexpensive and convenient food does so at a cost we'd like to avoid.

As a result of our discomfort, we look for other models that are closer to home, smaller scale, more accountable, and, we hope, more reflective of our own broader desires for a society that is more just, more ecologically sustainability, and more democratic. We think more about the physical design of our cities, how public policies promote (or get in the way of) healthier lifestyles, and whether we can regenerate more local and regional food systems as complements to, if not replacements for, the dominant food system. The question is to what extent these nascent local food systems can fulfill all of our desires – including giving us what we want, when we want it, and at a price we want to pay.

This book

This volume is a cross-disciplinary inquiry on topics relevant to local food system access, sustainability, and resilience. The contributions are from researchers working on social, ecological, political and ethical issues associated with food systems. Its focus is on the analysis of and lessons obtained from specific experiences relevant to local food systems, such as tapping urban farmers' markets to address issues of food access and public health, use of zoning to restrict the density of fast food restaurants in the hopes of reducing obesity rates in poorer neighborhoods, building a local food business to address twin problems of economic and nutritional distress, developing ways to reduce food waste and improve food access in poor urban neighborhoods, and asking whether the many, and diverse, hopes for urban agricultural are merited. There is enormous interest in urban and local food systems and production among policy-makers and citizens, with a wide array of policies and initiatives intended to increase food security, decrease ecological impacts, and improve public health. This collection is premised on the view that it is critical to conduct research on existing efforts to determine what works and to develop best practices in pursuit of sustainable and socially just urban food systems.

As such, the chapters in this volume focus on experiments, efforts to make the food system work for more people in urban America, especially those who are food insecure for whatever reason. Most were composed for a March 2015 workshop at Northeastern University in Boston, "Feeding Cities: Ethical and Policy Issues in Urban Food Systems." That workshop brought together an incredibly diverse group of nutritionists, urban planners, ethicists, agricultural economists, urban agriculture experts, sociologists and anthropologists, policy scholars, state and local government and non-profit officials, and, even, culinary experts, to discuss a broad array of topics oriented around three broad themes: expanding food security, building more sustainable local food systems, and ensuring food system resilience.

Part I: Ensuring food security

The five chapters in this part focus on broad issues of ensuring food security and health, particularly for lower-income populations with greater access to comparatively inexpensive, calorie-dense foods is than healthier options, with consequent impacts on their health.

We start by framing the very notion of "food security." What does that mean? Is it simply ensuring that people don't starve, or is it something more? In "Food security as a human rights issue," Sandra Raponi makes the argument for viewing – and acting – on food access in human rights terms, the idea that we all have a basic human right to adequate food that to date has not been taken seriously in the United States. The right to adequate food, she writes, is a right *to be able to feed oneself*, rather than simply a right to be fed. As such, Americans should advocate for policies that promote equitable access to food and that protect sustainable food security for current and future generations.

The conventional wisdom is that urban America is a barren landscape of food deserts, with far too many citizens lacking basic access to food sources. In "Population density, poverty, and food retail access in the United States," Wilde, Llobrera, and Ver Ploeg look at the retail food environment in the United States. Their empirical analysis shows that Americans living in densely populated urban areas actually have *higher* than average proximity to a supermarket, while those living in areas without a nearby supermarket tend to have high rates of automobile access. That leaves almost 5 percent of the population lacking *either* an automobile and a nearby supermarket. The implications of their empirical analysis include the need to look beyond simplistic notions of "food deserts" and focus as much on such factors as transportation. What good is a market if you cannot get to it?

Another bit of conventional wisdom is that low-income urban areas have a higher than average concentration of fast food restaurants, leading in turn to high obesity rates and other food-related health problems among low-income residents lacking healthier and affordable options. In "Super-sized strategies for improved health," Nelson and Banks take a close look at policies to restrict the density of fast food outlets through zoning, a strategy based on three assumptions: 1) closer proximity to fast food results in higher consumption; 2) higher consumption of fast food leads to weight gain; and 3) the weight gain from consuming fast food is bad for one's health and leads to poor health outcomes. They look at the case of South Los Angeles in particular and conclude that such zoning restrictions are likely to have minimal impact on obesity. Worse, they suggest, such efforts may have unintended consequences, including the perpetuation of spatially and socioeconomically stratified communities.

What about getting more affordable fresh fruits and vegetables closer to low-income and ethnically diverse populations? In "From food access to food justice," Shostak, Blum, Mancini, Oliveira, Robinson, and Satin-Hernandez review a pilot program in Somerville, Massachusetts, a densely populated small city just north of Boston. Somerville is home to three unique farmers' markets, including a mobile market that brings produce into low-income areas of the city. Here, they focus on the mobile market to show how locating markets in their community contexts highlights the multiple roles and functions of farmers' markets in urban areas. Different markets occupy specific niches, they argue, so it is critical that farmers are able to match their offerings to the demand at specific markets. Low-income consumers, for their part, can be active agents in determining the products made available to them, thereby advancing food justice.

What about those who are physically unable to get to markets due to age and disability? In "Farm to home," Ismail and Cuite review and assess a pilot program in New Brunswick, New Jersey that leveraged existing nutrition and "meals on wheels" programs to deliver fresh fruit and vegetables from a local farmers' market to homebound and low-income senior citizens. Their analysis of program successes and failures raises useful questions about food access and health. Is it simply enough to situate more markets near underserved populations if they cannot physically get there? What policy and administrative obstacles get in the way of greater access? Their ultimate goal is to get us to consider how local, urban food systems might be designed support the long-term nutritional needs of limited access populations. It won't be easy.

Part II: Building local food system sustainability

The chapters in this part focus on experiments in cultivating local food systems to act as complements to, if not substitutes for, the dominant food system. But these local food systems are more than about growing vegetables or creating incentives for consumers to buy local products. In many ways the next three chapters use a food system lens to cast a sometimes-uncomfortable gaze on broader issues of income, race and ethnicity, urban economic development, environmental justice, and sustainability in all of its meaning.

It is fitting that we start this part with a chapter on urban agriculture, a topic all the rage in cities across the country. But what is your urban agriculture for? In

"What grows in East New York," Daftary-Steel, Porter, Gervais, Vigil, and Marshall reflect on their experiences to address the many expectations – or dreams, if you will – placed on urban agriculture. In what they call "the unattainable trifecta of urban agriculture" they look at the myth that urban agriculture can, without long-term funding investments, simultaneously do three things that are each hard enough to do on their own: 1) provide good fresh food to people with limited financial resources at prices they can afford; 2) generate income for producers and create jobs funded by profits from sales; 3) provide job training, work experience, and/or leadership development for people typically excluded from employment. Based on their experiences, the authors address the challenges urban agriculture operations face in achieving these disparate goals, and what is needed to make this trifecta more attainable.

In a similar vein are efforts to catalyze local food systems and local economies through food hubs and other "incubators." In "Feeding community: A case study of a shared-use commercial kitchen in eastern Connecticut," Freake and Godfrey discuss lessons obtained so far in their effort to help small local farmers and low-income communities alike through a shared-use commercial kitchen. The facility in question is located in Willimantic, Connecticut, a once a thriving mill town that today has high poverty rates and a diverse population, with 40 percent identifying as Hispanic or Latino, beset with food security and health issues. Meanwhile, nearby small farms struggle for viability in a global food system where apples shipped in from New Zealand may be cheaper than those grown five miles away. To address these multiple needs, community members, including the authors, created CLiCK (Commercially Licensed Cooperative Kitchen), a non-profit, co-operative shared-use commercial and teaching kitchen to enable local farmers to add value to their products and extend their markets, entrepreneurs to incubate small-scale food businesses, and the whole community to benefit from healthy cooking and nutrition education classes. CLiCK has been designed to serve the needs of the community through its commitment to a just locally based sustainable and healthy food system. This chapter describes the long journey to CLiCK's creation, and its successes and struggles so far in meeting in multiple, not easily compatible goals.

The sustainability of food systems also depends on reducing their waste at multiple points in the food production, processing, consumption, and disposal life cycle. Can we do so *and* generate local economic gains *and* address issues of food access? In "Developing a food system-sensitive methodology to transform food 'waste,' create new food businesses, and address hunger in urban communities," O'Donnell, Deutsch, Yungmann, Zeitz, and Katz report on efforts in Philadelphia to address food waste at points in the food chain linking supermarkets to the public. They report on a pilot project connecting university researchers with business and charitable communities in an economically depressed area of the city. Their specific focus is on sustainable surplus-food management program designed to divert "surplus" fresh fruit and vegetables from the waste stream and return them to the economic/social food system through the creation of "value added" products that can be sold in local stores or donated to food pantries. Their experience shows how bringing together grocers and other food system experts, universities, communication specialists, environmental groups, and health experts can inform issues of food ethics and policy, and work to reduce food loss. In doing so, they also underscore how hard it is to maintain such initiatives in a system where the economic incentives to discard "surplus" food too often dominate.

Part III: Ensuring food system resilience

Finally, we want to know if local food systems broadly defined can be made more resilient in the face of disruption. The global food system has the virtue of being somewhat resilient insofar that interruptions in the supply of one particular commodity from one part of the world usually can be offset by suppliers elsewhere. After all, soybeans from Iowa are interchangeable with soybeans from Brazil, Canadian beef can substitute for American, and apples from New Zealand can take the place of apples from Washington State, or even Connecticut, if conditions warrant. But what about the tightly-coupled nature of local systems of food preparation and delivery? What are their points of potential system failure, and how should local policy-makers in particular reimagine these systems in light of insights obtained from resilience thinking?

Resilience includes safety. How safe are local food systems, particularly those serving at-risk populations? In "Food safety and the emergency food supply chain: Lessons from North Carolina food pantries," Chaifetz and Chapman examine a critical element in local food systems: food pantries. Food pantries play an outsized if incompletely understood role in meeting the needs of food-insecure population, but their supply chain and storage procedures are largely unregulated and understudied. Such issues may matter little for highly processed, shelf-stable foods, but are critical when it comes to fresh fruits and vegetables, dairy, and meat, components of healthier diets. Food pantries increasingly seek to supply such foods, but where do they get their supplies, how are these foods transported, and how are they stored before going to their intended recipients? Are those dependent on the emergency food system put at undue risk? In this chapter they examine the emergency food supply chain in North Carolina to assess points at which risks to food safety can emerge even as food panties try to plug gaps in the food supply. Overall, food pantries are diverse in their operations and capabilities. The results of their analysis provide a tool that food pantry managers can use to identify on-site risky supply chain behaviors and evaluate how to improve their systems.

Finally, what happens when the local food system gets hit by a disaster? How much food is available in your typical city, and how long might it take before the local system returns to normal? In "Creating a resilience assessment framework for urban food systems," Zeuli and Nijuis reflect on an effort by the city of Boston to assess its food system, identify points of vulnerability in food availability and access that could arise as a result of a natural disaster, and create a set of recommendations for implementation. Using a systems lens, they found some rather surprising, and disturbing, conditions: the long distances some foods take to get to Boston, the concentration of food distribution in a few places, some of them susceptible to flooding from climate change induced storm surges, the dependence of the local food system on a few roads, and the particular exposure of the emergency food system to system interruptions at the very moment it might be most needed. Their recommendations focus on integrating food system resilience thinking into urban policymaking and implementation, whether for future infrastructure development or to address the needs of at-risk populations.

As a group, the chapters in this volume offer lessons from real efforts to leverage local food systems in more equitable and sustainable ways. They also invite us to think more broadly about "local" food systems. It is one thing to advocate for the production of more local foods as a complement to the global food system. There is much to be gained, for all of us, in bringing back more vibrant local and regional food systems. But, as the various chapters here suggest, we all have much to do to make sure that the food system we want serves all of us.

Acknowledgements

Thanks to Northeastern University colleague Ronald Sandler for serving as co-organizer for the March 2015 "Feeding Cities" workshop from which this volume derives, to the College of Social Sciences and Humanities for financial support, to CSSH Assistant Dean Erika Koss in particular for her enthusiastic embrace of the Workshop and the overall efforts by the NU Consortium on Food Systems Sustainability, Health, and Equity to inculcate food systems thinking into our curriculum, to the staff of the School of Public Policy and Urban Affairs for their valuable logistical assistance, and, to all Workshop participants, whose contributions and engagement made the effort worthwhile. Thanks also to everyone at Routledge and, last but not least, to Claudia Larson, newly minted doctor of philosophy at Northeastern University, for her editorial help.

Notes

1 USDA, Food Expenditures, Table 7. Available online at www.ers.usda.gov/data-products/food-expenditures.aspx#.U3UFT17rVa/ (accessed May 30, 2016).
2 USDA, 2012 Census of Agriculture. Available online at www.agcensus.usda.gov/Publications/2012/Full_Report/Volume_1,_Chapter_1_US/st99_1_055_055.pdf (accessed May 30, 2016).

Part I

Ensuring food security

2 Food security as a human rights issue

Sandra Raponi

According to the United States Department of Agriculture (USDA), 14 percent of all U.S. households in 2014 experienced some level of food insecurity. This included 48.1 million adults and 7.9 million children (Coleman-Jensen et al. 2015). The number of food-insecure households increased significantly over the recent recession, from 11 percent of all households in 2008 to between 14 and 15 percent since. Despite this increase in apparent need, the U.S. Congress cut spending on the Supplemental Nutrition Assistance Program (SNAP), previously known as "food stamps," by $800 million in 2014, and by a total of $8.6 billion over the next decade. Even that cut was seen as a bit of a victory by program defenders, inasmuch as House Republicans initially sought closer to $40 billion in cuts.

In the United States, there has also been growing concern for food deserts, which the USDA defines as "urban neighborhoods and rural towns without ready access to fresh, healthy, and affordable food." It estimates that 23.5 million people in the United States live in food deserts (USDA a). This lack of access to nutritious food contributes to a poor diet and can lead to higher levels of obesity, diabetes, heart disease, and other diet-related illness.

Given these realities, why has more not been done in the United States to ensure sustainable food security? Unfortunately, despite the existence of some government programs like SNAP, providing food aid and ensuring food security has been largely viewed as a voluntary act of charity within the United States. In this chapter I argue that we should instead think of the failure of U.S. government to address the problem of food insecurity as a human rights issue (see also Raponi 2016). The right to adequate food is included as a human right in the *United Nations Declaration of Human Rights* (1948) and in the *International Covenant on Economic, Social and Cultural Rights* (1976). Many other international documents and institutions have affirmed and developed this right, including the UN Food and Agricultural Organization.

Appealing to the right to adequate food as it has been developed and applied internationally when addressing sustainable food security in urban areas within the United States is helpful for several reasons. First, being able to claim that one's human rights are being violated can be empowering for those who suffer from food insecurity. Second, given the normative weight of rights-discourse, appealing to the right to adequate food can have a powerful motivating force for activists, and it can increase political pressure on governments. Third, it is useful to draw on the work and progress that has been made by these international bodies, particularly in their assessment of the food policies of other countries. Fourth, it allows us to appeal to the international community for support as we push for reforms at home. In addition to using rights-language as a normative tool to promote food security, it is also important to advocate for legal protection of the right to adequate food and to support the ratification of the *International Covenant on Economic, Social and Cultural Rights*.

The right to adequate food in international law

Article 25 of the *United Nations Declaration of Human Rights* (1948) and Article 11.1 of the *International Covenant on Economic, Social, and Cultural Rights* (1976) protect the right to adequate food as part of the right to an adequate standard of living. The Covenant has been ratified by 164 state parties and signed by an additional five states. Although the United States has signed the Covenant, it is not legally binding on the United States because the U.S. Senate has not ratified it, as per requirements in the U.S. Constitution.

Article 11.2 of the Covenant affirms the *fundamental* right to be free from hunger. This right is considered to be more pressing since it involves ensuring that people do not die from hunger or suffer from malnutrition. Article 11.2 includes some guidance on how states should fulfill this right:

> State Parties ... recognizing the fundamental right of everyone to be free from hunger, shall take, individually and through international co-operation, the measures, including specific programmes, which are needed:
>
> (a) To improve methods of production, conservation and distribution of food by making full use of technical and scientific knowledge, by disseminating knowledge of the principles of nutrition and by developing or reforming agrarian systems in such a way as to achieve the most efficient development and utilization of natural resources;
> (b) Taking into account the problems of both food-importing and food-exporting countries, to ensure an equitable distribution of world food supplies in relation to need.

Article 11.2 suggests a comprehensive approach to preventing hunger that includes improving methods of production, conservation, distribution and the way resources are used, developing and investing in scientific and technical knowledge, educating the public about nutrition, and ensuring the equitable distribution of food in trade policies.

The right to food in international law is set at a minimal level as the right to *adequate* food, and is defined as food that is quantitatively and qualitatively adequate or sufficient for human beings to develop fully and maintain their physical and mental faculties. The Committee on Economic, Social, and Cultural

Rights and the UN Special Rapporteur on the Right to Adequate Food have provided guidance to countries on how to protect and fulfill this right. According to the Committee on Economic, Social, and Cultural Rights:

> the right to adequate food is realized when every man, woman and child, alone or in community with others, have the physical and economic access at all times to adequate food or means for its procurement ... [It requires the] availability of food in a quantity and quality sufficient to satisfy the dietary needs of individuals, free from adverse substances, and acceptable within a given culture [and] the accessibility of such food in ways that are sustainable.
> (General Comment 12, 1999)

It is common for people to interpret the right to adequate food as a right to be fed. However, providing food-insecure people with food or money to buy food is just one component of the right to adequate food; this right is primarily *a right to feed oneself* and to have access to food, rather than a right to be fed. This right is not only concerned with starvation and malnutrition, but also with food safety and sustainable food security.

The international right to adequate food also acknowledges the communal and cultural importance of food. Recognition of the communal importance of food can support the food sovereignty movement. Consequently, in addition to appealing to this international right to promote policies that increase access to food, we can also appeal to it in advocating for policies that protect food safety, promote nutrition and health, advance sustainable food practices, and support food sovereignty, as well as policies that are mindful of food's cultural and communal importance.

Many other international documents and institutions protect the right to adequate food, including the UN Food and Agricultural Organization (FAO). The *Universal Declaration on the Eradication of Hunger and Malnutrition* (1974) declares that "Every man, woman, and child has the inalienable right to be free from hunger and malnutrition in order to develop fully and maintain their physical and mental faculties." At the 1996 World Food Summit, the right to food was identified as central to achieving success against hunger and malnutrition. In the resulting Rome *Declaration on World Food Security*, governments affirmed "the right of everyone to have access to safe and nutritious food, consistent with the right to adequate food and the fundamental right of everyone to be free from hunger." Governments also agreed to take efforts to reduce the number of people suffering from hunger and malnutrition in half by 2015, based on the 1992 measurement of 840 million people. At the 2002 World Food Summit, the FAO adopted the *Right to Food Guidelines* to guide states in their implementation of the right to adequate food under the *Covenant on Economic, Social and Cultural Rights*.

The UN Millennium Development Goals adopted by nation states in 2000 included the goal to eradicate extreme poverty and hunger, and specifically to reduce the number of people suffering from hunger and malnutrition in half by

2015. While important progress has been made in the subsequent 15 years towards this target, there are still approximately 795 million undernourished people in the world, including more than 90 million children under the age of 5 (UN Millennium Goals Report 2015, p. 20). In 2015, states made a further commitment to "end hunger, achieve food security and improved nutrition, and promote sustainable agriculture" as part of the UN Sustainable Development Goals. The targets include ending hunger and all forms of malnutrition by 2030, and ensuring that all people have access to safe, nutritious and sufficient food all year round.

While the United States has undertaken international commitments to help reduce world hunger and malnutrition, it has avoided recognizing an enforceable "right" to adequate food either internationally or domestically. Before 2009, the United States simply voted against UN resolutions on the right to food. Under the Obama Administration, it voted in favor of UN resolutions on the right to food while stipulating that the United States rejects the idea that the right to food can be treated as an enforceable obligation (see Explanation by Huel 2009). The United States has also not provided legal and judicial protection of a right to adequate food, actions the FAO, the Committee on Economic, Social and Cultural Rights, and the Special Rapporteur on the Right to Food have deemed necessary. As the Special Rapporteur on the Right to Food, Hilal Elver, stated in her Interim Report to the General Assembly in 2014:

> While the right to food may once have been a controversial "positive" right, it is now enshrined in international law and States are obliged to ensure its progressive realization through ratification of international treaties and the development of supportive domestic and national legislation. However, many countries have failed to develop a judicial culture of recognition in practice, or the necessary legal frameworks required to ensure that the rights enshrined in the International Covenant on Economic, Social and Cultural Rights are justiciable. Accountability at both the international and national levels is paramount to ensuring that the right to food and its correlative obligations are being implemented ... States should enshrine the right to food in their domestic law, including through the constitution, and provide suitable mechanisms for effective redress in the event of violations of the right to food.
>
> (Elver 2014)

How can we draw upon these developments regarding the international right to food to promote food security in the United States?

Appealing to the right to adequate food to promote food security

The duty to respect the right to adequate food

International human rights law imposes three kinds of duties on nation states: to respect, to protect, and to fulfill human rights. The duty to respect a right primarily requires that governments and their agents do not interfere with a person's exercise of their rights. This is a comparatively low bar. The duties to protect and fulfill a right require positive action by the government, as well as resources. For example, states not only have a negative duty to respect the right to physical security by ensuring that state agents refrain from assaulting citizens; they also have a positive obligation to protect this right through a criminal justice system that includes police, courts, and prisons. Those who oppose recognizing a right to food as a human right are primarily concerned with the positive duties this would entail, rather than the more limited duty to not interfere with the right.

I begin with the negative duty to respect the right to adequate food since it is less controversial. We need to ask whether laws, policies and government actions interfere with a person's access to adequate food. First, consider legal restrictions on providing food to the hungry. Since January 2013, over 20 cities in the United States have enacted so-called "feeding bans," restrictions to prevent people from sharing food with homeless people (National Coalition for the Homeless Report 2014). These regulations constitute government interference with a person's ability to access food. For example, Arnold Abbott, a 90-year-old chef who runs a nonprofit group that has been distributing food in city parks in Fort Lauderdale for over 20 years was charged in October 2014 for violating a recent city ordinance that restricts sharing food outdoors (Barkley 2014). The legal penalty for violating this ordinance was a $500 fine or 60 days in prison for each charge. He was charged multiple times. At trial, Abbott argued that the law violated his religious freedom. The case gained widespread media attention and led to protests against the city of Fort Lauderdale. Others also filed suits against the city, claiming that the law violated their First Amendment right to free speech. In December 2014, a Florida Circuit Court temporarily halted the ordinance and directed all parties involved to reach a compromise through mediation. These cases are still ongoing (Swanson 2016). While such laws target the ability of people to provide food to the hungry, the effect of the law is that of limiting people's access to food that would have otherwise been available to them. One can see this more clearly when one considers what happened in Abbott's case. The police officers literally threw the food Abbott had prepared into garbage bins as those who had waited in line for the food looked on.

Some of these laws seem particularly problematic because they appear to be part of growing attempts to criminalize the homeless and to reduce their visibility. But what if regulations about distributing food to others are genuinely motivated by the goal of ensuring food safety? For example, many states and cities have regulations regarding what kind of food can be donated to food pantries and emergency kitchens, such as requiring food to be pre-packaged and labeled. In such cases, the goal of not limiting access to food has to be weighed against the goal of ensuring food safety, which is another component of the right to adequate food. In a court hearing on South Carolina's food-sharing ban, the argument that the law's purpose was food safety was challenged by the state's ACLU chapter. It pointed out that similar restrictions were not being applied to family reunions or food-sharing events in the park, and that there had not been any cases of a homeless person getting sick (Levintova 2014).

Second, consider local bylaws that restrict one's ability to produce food, especially in urban and residential areas. If a local government restricts or bans community gardens, this constitutes government interference with people's ability to access adequate food. If a local government unduly restricts gardens on residential properties or bans certain food producing practices in residential areas, such as not permitting backyard hens, this also may constitute government interference with people's ability to have access to affordable and nutritious food. While there may be good reasons to restrict certain forms of food production in densely populated urban areas, especially if there is a concern about public health, this is an argument that would need to be proven in order to justify restricting people's access to adequate food. In the case of backyard hens, such concerns are often exaggerated, as demonstrated by the experience of cities that permit this (Beyko 2012).

In Canada, people have argued that city prohibitions on backyard hens violate their right to food under the *Universal Declaration of Human Rights* and the *International Covenant of Economic, Social and Cultural Rights* (Davis 2012). In one case, *R v. Hughes*, the accused was charged with violating Calgary's bylaw by keeping chickens in the backyard of his residential property. Unfortunately he was not able to establish that this restriction violated the rights and freedoms protected in the *Canadian Charter of Rights and Freedoms,* which does not include a right to adequate food, and the Court did not consider his argument that the law violated the *Universal Declaration of Human Rights* (Beyko 2012).

Despite this loss in court, food activists and locavores have been able to persuade local governments to allow backyard hens at least in part by appealing to the right to adequate food. They have also argued that removing restrictions on home gardens and hens promotes environmental sustainability by increasing access to locally produced food (Schindler 2012: 2). For example, the zoning ordinance of Cherokee County, Georgia explains that "[t]he keeping of hens supports a local, sustainable food system by providing an affordable, nutritious food source of fresh eggs" (Salkin 2011). Over 166 cities in the U.S. allow chickens in residential areas, including Austin, Boston, Nashville, St. Louis, Tulsa, New York, Seattle, Portland, Houston and San Francisco, and changes have been proposed in other cities, including Albany, Lafayette in Colorado, and North Salt Lake in Utah (Salkin 2011; Beyko 2012). In Canada, a number of cities allow backyard hens, including Vancouver, Victoria, Niagara Falls, Brampton, and Guelph while other municipalities are undergoing pilot projects (Beyko 2012).

The duty to protect the right to adequate food from external interferences

Just as the government has a duty to protect our physical security against interferences from other people, we can argue that the government should similarly protect our right to adequate food against interferences by others. This seems particularly important in the case of the right to adequate food when we consider how government laws and policies regarding agriculture, commerce, zoning laws, foreign trade, and economic strategies can affect people's ability to acquire adequate food.

Governments can set laws and policies to prevent people from being deprived of their right to adequate food. For example, consider the case of landowners who have traditionally used their land to grow crops that meet the nutritional needs of the local population but then decide to grow different kinds of crops for export to other countries for greater economic gain (see also Shue 1990). If they make this change, the food supply for the local population will diminish and food will be less affordable. A government may discourage or prevent this through trade agreements, subsidies, incentives, or disincentives. A clearer case is that of a factory that is contaminating the food supply of a local community. By restricting the actions of the polluters, the government can protect people's access to safe food. In these scenarios, people previously had access to safe and affordable food but the actions of others have interfered with their ability to enjoy this right.

The right to adequate food also includes protecting sustainable food security in the future. This can be addressed by government restrictions on agricultural practices and products that contribute to soil erosion or reduce the ability to grow food crops in the future. A government can protect the right to adequate food by prohibiting or restricting the use of certain pesticides, monocropping practices, and certain genetically modified (GM) crops with problematic agricultural or ecological impacts.

How might the right to adequate food be applied to food deserts, rural and urban areas where people do not have ready access to affordable, fresh and nutritious food? The USDA's Economic Research Service estimates that 23.5 million people in the United States live in food deserts. More than half of these people are low-income. In the case of urban food deserts, many of these are located in poor areas that have lost nearby farms over the years due to urbanization and large industrial farming. These areas have also lost small local food markets over the years as larger supermarkets have grown in more economically viable suburban areas. These communities may only have nearby access to unhealthy fast food restaurants and convenience stores that offer few healthy and affordable food options. This lack of access to affordable nutritious food contributes to poor diet and can lead to higher levels of obesity and other diet-related diseases, such as diabetes and heart disease. This is a problem that properly falls under the right to adequate food since this right includes having access to food that is quantitatively and qualitatively sufficient for human beings to develop fully and maintain their physical and mental faculties.

Local governments can protect people's access to nutritious food through permits and zoning bylaws. For example, they can limit the amount of unhealthy fast food restaurants in these areas, and they can provide subsidies and incentives to nearby grocery stores. Unfortunately regulation is only a small component of what is required to address these problems; governments must also take positive action and invest resources. Restricting the number of fast food restaurants will not be effective unless there is also an increase in affordable healthy food, including prepared foods. In addition to permitting and not interfering with the development of farmers' markets on public property, mobile grocery vendors, and community gardens, we can argue that public funds should to be used to support these ventures so they are more accessible to low-income communities. *Protecting* access to food in poor urban areas requires policies that prevent food deserts from developing. But once food deserts have already developed, more is needed to *fulfill* the right to adequate food.

The duty to fulfill the right to adequate food

The duty to fulfill the right to adequate food requires additional government action and resources. Providing SNAP benefits or food stamps to low-income families is a clear example of this. In the case of urban food deserts, investing in affordable and efficient public transportation can also increase access to affordable, healthy food. Recent studies have suggested that reducing unhealthy fast food restaurants and adding grocery stores in urban food deserts do not automatically lead to significant improvements in people's diets (Cummins et al. 2014). Moreover, while the right to adequate food has traditionally been understood to mean having physical or economic access to food that is adequate for a healthy diet, simply making healthy food more available does not seem to be sufficient in the case of low-income communities; more needs to be done to change people's behavior. Government programs that promote healthy eating may also be needed, particularly programs that develop healthy eating habits in schools.

More importantly, we also need to understand the connection between food-related illnesses and poverty. In urban areas in the United States, people who are food-insecure also typically have low incomes. Recent studies have shown that members of low-income and food-insecure families may suffer from high levels of stress, anxiety and depression. High levels of stress, anxiety and depression have been linked to weight gain and obesity (Food Research and Action Center 2015). Families may not feel they have the time or energy to shop for groceries and prepare healthy meals. Unhealthy fast food may be seen as easy comfort food. These families may not have the time or energy for physical activity. Simply providing people SNAP benefits and easier access to grocery stores will not address these other factors. It is difficult to effectively fulfill the right to adequate food without also fulfilling the broader right to an adequate standard of living. In this regard, it is important to remember that the right to food in the *Universal Declaration of Human Rights* and in the *International Covenant of Economic, Social and Cultural Rights* is not a stand-alone right; instead, it is part of the broader right to an adequate standard of living.

Objections, and responses to them

Why is there so much resistance in the United States to recognizing a right to adequate food? Elsewhere, I focus on the philosophical and practical objections that have been raised against recognizing the right to adequate food as a human right (Raponi 2016). One important objection is that fulfilling the right to adequate food is not feasible for all countries, particularly poor ones. How can we say that nation states have an obligation to secure this right if it is not possible for all to do so? A second objection is that the right to adequate food is not justiciable and cannot be legally protected because doing so would require courts to engage in resource allocation, and this is a matter that is best left to elected policymakers.

While it is true that nations cannot be obligated to do what is not feasible for them to do, we can still ask what a given society *can* do to secure the enjoyment of certain rights *as much as possible* (Pogge 1995: 118). The fulfillment of the rights protected in the *International Covenant of Social and Cultural Rights* is measured according to a progressive standard. According to the *ICESCR*, nation states must take steps towards the fulfillment of these rights to the maximum extent possible *given their available resources*. Article 2.1 of the ICESCR states:

> Each State Party to the present Covenant undertakes to take steps ... to the maximum of its available resources, with a view to achieving progressively the full realization of the rights recognized in the present Covenant by all appropriate means, including particularly the adoption of legislative measures.

When the Committee evaluates a state's compliance with the treaty, it considers whether a state could do more but is simply unwilling to do so, or whether the state is not able to do more given its limited resources.

In support of the second objection, critics claim that securing the right to food and other subsistence rights requires courts to engage in questions of budget allocation and program development that are best left to other branches of government. They argue that courts lack the institutional capacity and democratic legitimacy to determine such matters. How much should be spent to secure access to adequate food, housing, health care, social assistance, and education? What are the best ways to secure these rights? While the role of judges in addressing these questions is limited, courts can nonetheless determine when the government is not doing enough to fulfill the right to adequate food. Judges can also provide some guidance regarding what kinds of action would better meet the government's obligations, given its available resources. If many people are malnourished in a relatively wealthy country, this is an indication that the government needs to be doing more to address this problem. A government can still have a significant amount of flexibility regarding how to address the court's concerns.

Many countries have in fact protected the right to food as a legal right. Twenty-three countries have constitutional protection for the right to food (Knuth and Vidar 2011). Five states recognize the right to food as part of the right to an adequate or dignified standard of living. In 33 countries, the right to food is implicit in a broader human right, such as a right to basic needs. Thirteen countries recognize the right to adequate food as a policy directive. In some states, courts have recognized this right in their interpretation of other constitutional rights (Knuth and Vidar 2011). In India and Ireland, for example, courts have protected the right to food as falling under a constitutional right to life. In *Kishen Pattnayak & Antother v. State of Orissa* (1989) and *People's Union for Civil Liberties v.*

Union of India & Others (2001), the Supreme Court of India recognized the right to food under the right to life guaranteed under Article 21 of the Indian Constitution. In *G v. An Bord Uchtala and Others* (1980), the Irish Supreme Court stated that the right to life in Article 40 of the Irish Constitution necessarily implies "the right to preserve and defend, and to have preserved and defended that life and the right to maintain that life at a proper human standard in matters of food, clothing and habitation" (Knuth and Vidar 2011). The Committee on Economic, Social, Cultural Rights and the Special Rapporteur on the Right to Food have argued that domestic courts should interpret the right to life as including the right to food if there is no other legal protection for this right. Some scholars have argued that American courts can and should do this as well (Sunstein 2005).

It is helpful to consider how courts in other countries have adjudicated the right to adequate food. In *People's Union for Civil Liberties v. Union of India & Others*, the Supreme Court of India determined a minimal level for basic nutrition and it appointed commissioners to monitor implementation of its interim orders. These interim orders led to new and better government programs, such as mid-day meals for school children, food entitlements in child care centers, and subsidized food for specific vulnerable groups (Knuth and Vidar 2011).

Although there is no federal constitutional protection of the right to adequate food and other socio-economic rights in the United States, we can find legal protection for other socio-economic rights in the constitutions of some U.S. states, including the right to education, housing, welfare assistance, health care, and labor rights. Many U.S. state constitutions require that the state government establish and support public schools and that they provide a "sound" basic education. In terms of labor rights, many state constitutions address the number of hours in a legal workday, workers' compensation, and wage issues, and require that the government ensure safe working conditions. Zackin (2013: 110) argues that proponents of labor rights sought to "create obligations on government to intervene, placing itself between employers and laborers, and providing protection from the often brutal conditions market capitalism had created."

Consequently, American courts have already been adjudicating cases involving social-economic rights and rights that require state intervention. Take one state, New York, as a case. In *Campaign for Fiscal Equity v. State of New York* (2001), the New York Court of Appeals determined that the State of New York breached its constitutional duties by not providing a sound high school level education to all students, regardless of their economic situation. It ordered the state government to ensure that every school in New York City had the resources necessary to provide the opportunity for a sound basic education, and it ordered that a system of accountability be put in place (Albisa and Sculz 2008: 242). In another instance, the New York Court of Appeals found that the state had a positive duty "to provide welfare payments to anyone considered indigent under the state's 'need standard,' even if the individual could not present papers proving that he or she received no support from relatives" (*Tucker v. Toia* 1977). In a series of cases beginning in 1975, the New York Supreme Court recognized a right to shelter based on general welfare provisions in the State's constitutions and other statutes. In its reasons, it also supported a right to food: "There cannot be the slightest doubt that shelter, along with food, are the most basic human needs" (*Township of Mount Laurel* 1975). The Court held that a zoning ordinance violated the right to adequate housing for all because it excluded low- and moderate-income families. It granted the township 90 days to reform its land use regulations. When the township failed to do so, the Court required that each municipality prove the likelihood that lower-income housing would be constructed and it set up a panel of three judges to assess the process (*Township of Mount Laurel* 1983). This action led to state passage of its Fair Housing Act in 1985 and the creation of a Council on Affordable Housing to monitor compliance (Albisa and Schultz 2008: 245).

Based on such cases, Albisa and Schultz conclude that courts do have the capacity to assess the availability of resources, to balance the competing demands on those resources, and to monitor the adequacy of complex social policies (Albisa and Schultz 2008: 247). As these cases illustrate, while a court of law may not be the best institution to monitor compliance on an ongoing basis, it can require that a government create other procedures and administrative bodies to monitor compliance and ensure accountability.

Conclusion: why the right to adequate food matters

Rather than relying on a government's charitable good will to ensure food security, it is essential to advocate for laws that protect the right to adequate food. Legal and judicial protection of the right to food in other countries has led to government accountability and increased food security. In addition, it gives people who are food-insecure an avenue of recourse against their government. In the United States, legal and judicial protection of other socio-economic rights has also led to government accountability and increased protection. In the absence of legislation, bringing cases before the courts can still be useful. Some courts may be open to extending existing legal protection for social-economic rights to include the right to adequate food.

In the absence of legal and judicial protection, appealing to the right to adequate food can still be politically effective given the significant normative weight of the idea of human rights. Arguing that a government is violating people's international right to adequate food can put pressure on governments to ensure food security, and it can also help gain public support. Advocates can also appeal to the international community for support. For example, when the City of Detroit cut off water from poor residents who were unable to afford an increase in their water bills, the residents argued that the City had violated their right to water under international law. Two UN experts, the Special Rapporteur on the human right to water and the Special Rapporteur on the right to adequate housing, investigated these cases and urged the City to restore access to citizens who are unable to pay their bills. They stated that failure to do this would constitute a violation of the most basic human rights and they called for the establishment of a mandatory federal water and sewerage affordability standard along with the introduction of special policies and tailored support for people in particularly vulnerable circumstances (UN News Centre 2014). In response to protests and widespread criticism, Detroit began a Water Residential Assistance Program for low-income residents. Priority is given to residents with past-due accounts who are at risk of having their water shut off.

In an interview, the former Special Rapporteur on the Right to Food, Oliver De Schutter, was asked about the how the idea of the right to food has helped to address hunger. He responded:

> In 1996 we had a pivotal moment at the United Nations World Food Summit in Rome: for the first time the idea of the right to food was identified as central to achieving successes against hunger and malnutrition. Out of that meeting, many governments requested that human rights bodies develop the normative concept of the right to food. Until then the concept was mostly just a slogan, seen as abstract and vague—sympathetic but not useful. Now the idea has become operational. It is increasingly seen as essential to fighting hunger: unless you increase political pressure on governments, unless you ensure that those in need participate in identifying the solutions to the obstacles they face and play an active role in monitoring progress, nothing will change. This is a core idea of the right to food. It is based on the recognition that you cannot work for people without people
>
> (Lappé 2011).

References

Albisa, C., and Schultz, J. 2008. "The United States: A Ragged Patchwork." In Malcolm Langford (ed.), *Social Rights Jurisprudence: Emerging Trends in International and Comparative Law*. Cambridge University Press, 230–249.

Barkley, E. 2014. "Florida Activist Arrested for Serving Food to Homeless." *National Public Radio*, November 6. Available online at www.npr.org/blogs/thesalt/2014/11/06/362019133/florida-activists-arrested-for-serving-food-to-homeless (accessed September 7, 2016).

Beyko, H. 2012. "Fowl Play? A Look into Recent Canadian Reform Efforts for Backyard Chicken Legislation." ABlawg: The University of Calgary Faculty of Law Blog. September 19, 2012. Available online at http://ablawg.ca/wp-content/uploads/2012/09/Blog_HB_Backyard_Chickens_Sept2012.pdf (accessed September 7, 2016).

Coleman-Jensen, A., Rabbitt, M., Gregory, C., and Singh, A. 2015. "Household Food Security in the United States in 2014." USDA Economic Research Service.

Cummins, S., Flint, E., and Matthews, S. 2014. "New Neighborhood Grocery Store Increased Awareness of Food Access but Did Not Alter Dietary Habits or Obesity." *Health Affairs* 33.2: 283–291.

Davis, A. 2012. "Is Keeping Hens in the City a Charter Right?" *Macleans*, March 12, 2012.

International Human Rights Clinic. 2013. *Nourishing Change: Fulfilling the Right to Food in the United States*. NYU School of Law.

Knuth, L., and Vidar, M. 2011. "Constitutional and Legal Protection of the Right to Food around the World." U.N. Food and Agriculture Organization. Available online at www.fao.org/docrep/016/ap554e/ap554e.pdf (accessed September 7, 2016).

Lappé, A. 2011. "Who Says Food is a Human Right": Olivier De Schutter, the UN's Special Rapporteur on the Right to Food, Makes the Case in this Q&A." *The Nation.* September 14, 2011.

Levintova, H. 2014. "Is Giving Food to the Homeless Illegal in Your City Too?" *Mother Jones.* Available online at www.motherjones.com/politics/2014/11/90-year-old-florida-veteran-arrested-feeding-homeless-bans (accessed September 7, 2016).

Pogge, T. 1995. "How Should Human Rights be Conceived?" *Jahrbuch fur Recht und Ethik* 3: 103–120.

Raponi, S. 2016. "A Defense of the Human Right to Adequate Food." *Res Publica.* Forthcoming.

Salkin, P. 2011. "Feeding the Locavores, One Chicken at a Time: Regulating Backyard Chickens." *Zoning and Planning Law Report*, 34.3.

Schindler, S. 2012. "Of Backyard Chickens and Front Yard Gardens: The Conflict between Local Governments and Locavores." *Tulane Law Review* 87.2.

Shue, H. 1980. *Basic Rights*. Princeton: Princeton University Press.

Sunstein, C. 2005. "Why Does the American Constitution Lack Social and Economic Guarantees?" In Michael Ignatieff (ed.), *American Exceptionalism*. Princeton University Press, 90–110.

Swanson, J. 2015. "One Year after Outcry, Groups Are Still Feeding Homeless despite Ban." *New Times Broward Palm Beach.* October 15, 2015.

United Nations News Centre. 2014. "In Detroit, City-Backed Water Shut-Offs Contrary to Human Rights, Say UN Experts." Available online at www.un.org/apps/news/story. asp?NewsID=49127#.VTMkb0vOAgI (accessed September 7, 2016).

Zackin, E. 2013. *Looking for Rights in All the Wrong Places: Why State Constitutions Contain America's Positive Rights*. Princeton University Press.

Documents and cases

Agricultural Act of 2014, H.R. 2642; Public Law 113-79 of the 113th Congress.

Campaign for Fiscal Equity v. State of New York, 100 N.Y. 2d 893 (2003).

City of Johannesburg and Others v. Lindiwe Mazibuko and Others, Case CCR 39/09 ZACC 28.

Committee on Economic, Social and Cultural Rights, General Comment 12, Right to Adequate Food (Twentieth session, 1999), U.N. Doc. E/C.12/1999/5 (1999).

Explanation of Position by Craig Kuehl, United States Advisor, on Resolution L.30, Rev. 1 – The Right to Food, in the Third Committee of the Sixty-Fourth Session of the United Nations General Assembly (November 19, 2009). Available online at http://usun.state. gov/remarks/4560 (accessed September 7, 2016).

Food and Agriculture Organization of the United Nations. The State of Food Insecurity in the World 2014. Available online at www.fao.org/3/a-i4030e.pdf (accessed September 7, 2016).

Food Research and Action Center, Understanding the Connection between Food Insecurity and Obesity. October 15, 2015.

G v. An Bord Uchtala and Others [1980] IR 32.

Gosselin v. Quebec (Attorney General) [2002] 4 S.C.R. 429, 2002 SCC 84.

Interim Report of the Special Rapporteur on the Right to Food, Hilal Elver, Submitted to the General Assembly. Sixty-Ninth Session. A/67/275 (August 7, 2014).

International Covenant on Economic, Social, and Cultural Rights (1976).

Kishen Pattnayak & Another v. State of Orissa (S.C. 1989).

National Coalition for the Homeless Report. Share No More: The Criminalization of Efforts to Feed People In Need. 2014. Available online at http://nationalhomeless.org/wp-content/uploads/2014/10/Food-Sharing2014.pdf (accessed September 7, 2016).

People's Union for Civil Liberties v. Union of India & Others (S.C. 2001).

Rome Declaration on World Food Security. 1996. FAO. Available online at www.fao.org/wfs/index_en.htm (accessed September 7, 2016).

Southern Burlington County N.A.A.C.P. v. Township of Mount Laurel, 67 N.J. 151 (1975).

Southern Burlington County N.A.A.C.P. v. Township of Mount Laurel, 92 N.J. 205 (1983).

Tucker v. Toia 43 N.Y.2d 1, 7 (1977).

Universal Declaration on the Eradication of Hunger and Malnutrition (1974).

United Nations Declaration of Human Rights (1948).

United Nations, *The Millennium Development Goals Report, 2015*.

United States Department of Agriculture (a). Food Deserts. Available online at http://apps.ams.usda.gov/fooddeserts/foodDeserts.aspx (accessed October 15, 2013).

United States Department of Agriculture (b). Food Security of U.S. Households in 2013. Available online at www.ers.usda.gov/topics/food-nutrition-assistance/food-security-in-the-us/key-statistics-graphics.aspx#foodsecure (accessed September 7, 2016).

3 Population density, poverty, and food retail access in the United States[1,2]

An empirical approach

Parke Wilde, Joseph Llobrera, and Michele Ver Ploeg

The United States in recent years has faced public concerns about unhealthy eating patterns, low consumption of fruits and vegetables, high rates of overweight and obesity, and household food insecurity. These concerns have generated a lively policy debate about the adequacy of the food retail environment, especially in low-income areas, and whether and how public policy could intervene to improve the retail environment in underserved areas (USDA Economic Research Service 2009; Rose 2010; Gittelsohn and Lee 2013).

These policy discussions have led to research that has attempted to define which areas may be underserved and have inadequate food retail. Such areas sometimes have been called "food deserts," although use of this term may be declining. Informally, the term "food desert" may be used to describe neighborhoods that lack healthy food resources. More formally, USDA's Economic Research Service classifies a census tract that meets a particular definition of low income and distance from the nearest supermarket as a "food desert" (Economic Research Service 2013). To understand the implications of alternative definitions, this study describes and compares three approaches that have been used to identify geographic areas with inadequate food retail:

- a *low-income low-access approach*, which identifies geographic areas that are low-income and lack a supermarket within a specified distance;
- a *low-vehicle low-access approach*, which identifies geographic areas that have low rates of vehicle access and lack a supermarket within a specified distance;
- a *relative distance approach*, which identifies geographic areas that have worse-than-usual proximity to a supermarket, compared with other neighborhoods that have similar population density and vehicle access rates.

These three approaches have been used in research applications and widely-circulated online tools. A low-income low-access approach was the primary approach used in USDA's online food desert atlas and still is one approach used in an updated version of this online tool, called the Food Access Research Atlas (FARA) (Economic Research Service 2013). A newer low-vehicle low-access approach also is used in the updated online FARA tool (Economic Research

Service 2013). A relative distance approach has been used in the definition of areas with limited supermarket access (LSA) by The Reinvestment Fund, one of several notable non-governmental research initiatives using alternative definitions of adequacy (The Reinvestment Fund 2011).

These tools are important because they may be used as inputs to policy decisions about subsidies or tax breaks to encourage retailers to locate in underserved locations or zoning rules to guide retailer location choices. However, retailers' location decisions respond primarily to market incentives rather than policy initiatives. Food retailers choose locations that they judge will be profitable. The profitability of a particular location depends on (a) the number and buying power of potential customers in nearby residential neighborhoods, (b) the nature of competition from other retailers, and (c) land, labor, and capital costs, which vary from place to place. Retailers cannot afford to build supermarkets in locations with too few customers or too many competitors.

The three research approaches lead to distinct conclusions about the adequacy of food retail conditions nationally and about which particular geographic areas lack adequate retail. Although they have similar purposes, the approaches differ in the underlying household-level circumstance or condition that motivates the methodology; they differ in implicit assumptions about the relationships between poverty, vehicle access, population density, and proximity to supermarkets; and they differ in their method for aggregating data from basic units (such as a census block group) to larger geographic units (such as a census tract).

This study compares and contrasts the three approaches using a common data source, a representative random sample of more than 33,000 census block groups in the continental United States. A census block is the smallest geographic unit used by the U.S. Census Bureau, while a census block group is a subdivision of a census tract that generally contains between 600 and 3,000 people (U.S. Census). Using this data source, we address four empirical questions about characteristics of small geographic areas (census block groups):

1 What is the empirical relationship between poverty and proximity to supermarkets?
2 What is the empirical relationship between population density and proximity to supermarkets?
3 What is the empirical relationship between vehicle access and proximity to supermarkets?
4 What is the average proximity to a supermarket for geographic areas with particular levels of population density and vehicle access rates?

These concrete empirical questions are important for two reasons. First, the basic relationships among poverty, population density, vehicle access, and proximity to supermarkets are interesting in their own right; in some cases, these relationships are surprising and contradict the conventional wisdom. Second, these empirical questions help in making choices among the three research approaches and in developing improved methods for identifying areas with inadequate food retail access.

This study contributes to a research literature that also includes several other important lines of work. The three approaches here focus on proximity to supermarkets, using retailer data that are available at the national level, while other research addresses different retail formats, including healthy food initiatives in smaller stores, using retailer data that are only available in particular locations (Gittelsohn, Rowan, and Gadhoke 2012). The three approaches used here focus on the nearest supermarket, while other research measures distances to potentially more distant retailers patronized by food consumers (USDA Economic Research Service 2012; Apparicio, Cloutier, and Shearmur 2007; Cole 1997). The three approaches used here merely describe food retail conditions, while other research seeks to measure the relationship of these conditions to diet and health outcomes (Gibson 2011; Leung, et al. 2011; Chen, Florax, and Snyder 2010). For this study, it was sufficient to better understand the geographic conditions and computational methods in high-profile online tools that are used to identify areas with inadequate proximity to the nearest supermarket.

Background

The USDA has published two reports measuring access to affordable and nutritious food nationwide (USDA Economic Research Service 2009; USDA Economic Research Service 2012). Retail access conditions depend to a large extent on competition in economic markets. An earlier literature in economics paid close attention to the relationship between the number of retailers in a particular area and their degree of market power (Fik 1988; Benson and Faminow 1985; Cotterill 1986). A line of research tracing back to Huff (1964) considered the question of how large each retailer's catchment area would be if consumers sought to shop at the closest retailer. In part responding to changes in the diversity of retail formats, some more recent research has focused on the relationship between market power and the mix of services that retailers offer (Bonanno and Lopez 2009).

This type of economic analysis adds new insight to existing lines of research on inadequate food retail access. For example, Broda, Leibtag, and Weinstein (2009) note that low-income consumers differ from other consumers not only in their more frequent use of small retailers (which may have higher food prices and locations close to home) but also in their more frequent use of superstores or supercenters (which may have lower food prices and locations farther from home). Bitler and Haider (2011) discuss both the supply and demand for food retail services, recognizing that in some cases it is a market equilibrium outcome to have only a small number of retailers in a particular geographic area.

This study focuses on three high-profile existing approaches to identifying geographic locations with inadequate supermarket access. The three approaches differ in their implicit assumption about the underlying household-level condition that is most important.

The low-income low-access approach. In an online mapping tool and accompanying data resources, USDA's Food Access Research Atlas (FARA) identifies census tracts as having inadequate food retail if they meet both a low-income definition and a low-access definition (Economic Research Service 2013).

- *Low-income* tracts satisfy an absolute poverty standard or a relative income standard. The absolute standard is having a poverty rate of at least 20 percent, based on the federal government's poverty guideline, which is a fixed national threshold. The relative standard is having census-tract median income at or below 80 percent of the median income in the corresponding metropolitan area or (for non-metropolitan areas) the entire state. This second standard varies across geographic locations.
- *Low-access* tracts have at least a third of the population or at least 500 people with low access. Low-access, for ERS, means low proximity to the nearest supermarket, defined using a different distance threshold in urban areas (at least 1 mile from a supermarket) and rural areas (at least 10 miles from a supermarket).

In this approach to classifying census tracts, some complexity arises from the need to aggregate up to the census-tract level, but the implicit underlying concept is clear. A person qualifies as having inadequate food retail access if he or she is low-income (based on having income below either the poverty line or 80 percent of area median income) and lives farther than the threshold distance from the nearest supermarket (where the threshold distance is 1 mile in urban areas and 10 miles in rural areas). This approach does not explicitly refer to vehicle access, but both the low-income standard and the distinction between urban and rural areas may be motivated by concern for those who lack either an automobile or a nearby supermarket.

The low-vehicle low-access approach

USDA's FARA tool recently has added more information so that an alternative vehicle-based measure can be constructed. A tract is identified as having low vehicle availability "if more than 100 households in the tract have no vehicle available and are more than 0.5 miles from the nearest supermarket" (Economic Research Service 2013).

The relative distance approach

The Reinvestment Fund (TRF), a non-governmental organization prominent in community food security research, identifies areas with limited supermarket access (LSA). Like USDA, TRF makes the results available in a popular online mapping tool. TRF uses a relative distance-to-supermarket concept somewhat akin to a relative income threshold in poverty measurement. A particular block group has low relative access if its distance to the nearest supermarket is longer than a threshold distance, which varies across 13 comparison-group strata, defined by combinations of population density and vehicle access rates.

For each comparison-group stratum, the threshold distance for determining whether the block group has limited access is based on the distance to the nearest supermarket for higher-income block groups in the stratum that are presumably not deprived. TRF computes the benchmark distance as the median distance to the nearest supermarket for those block groups with higher income (based on area median income above 120 percent of median income for the metropolitan area or state). Several findings are useful for understanding TRF's concept of inadequacy:

- The four rural strata with the lowest population density have 11.7 percent of the U.S. population. All of these strata have high vehicle access in TRF's classification. In these strata, the adequate benchmark distance ranges from 5.5 miles to 17.5 miles. This distance is roughly comparable to the 10-mile threshold used by USDA's FARA in rural areas.
- The five urban strata with the highest population density have 50.3 percent of the U.S. population. All but one of these strata have medium or high vehicle access in TRF's classification. In these strata, the adequate benchmark distance ranges from 0.15 miles to 1 mile.
- Only 1 of the 13 strata has low vehicle access in TRF's classification. It has a high population density and represents 6.6 percent of the U.S. population. Its adequate benchmark distance is just 0.29 miles.

In TRF's approach, the threshold distance varies across the comparison-group strata. For some locations, the threshold distance is larger than 5 miles, recognizing that many residents have vehicles. In other locations, the threshold for inadequate retail access may be as small as 0.15 miles or 0.29 miles, which is shorter than the threshold distance to supermarket used in other approaches with which we are familiar. With such small threshold distances, many locations may be classified as having inadequate access.

Conclusions about retail adequacy for census tracts necessarily build on conclusions about retail adequacy for smaller geographic units. In very small geographic areas, such as a census block group or a 1-km or 0.5-km grid square, the research literature generally treats resident households as if they share the same food retail environment. Building on the identification of small geographic units where households have inadequate access, one can determine which larger geographic areas (such as census tracts or counties) have sufficient numbers of such households or individuals to qualify as areas with limited supermarket access. For these larger geographic units, it is clear that research methods must acknowledge the internal heterogeneity in food retail access.

Conclusions about retail adequacy in small geographic units necessarily build on a concept of adequacy at the household level. It is useful to make this household-level concept explicit rather than having readers derive it implicitly from definitions of adequacy for geographic areas. To define adequacy at the level of the household, much of the literature focuses on the presence of supermarkets within a specified threshold distance from home. A sensible threshold distance may depend on whether a household has a vehicle. A common threshold distance

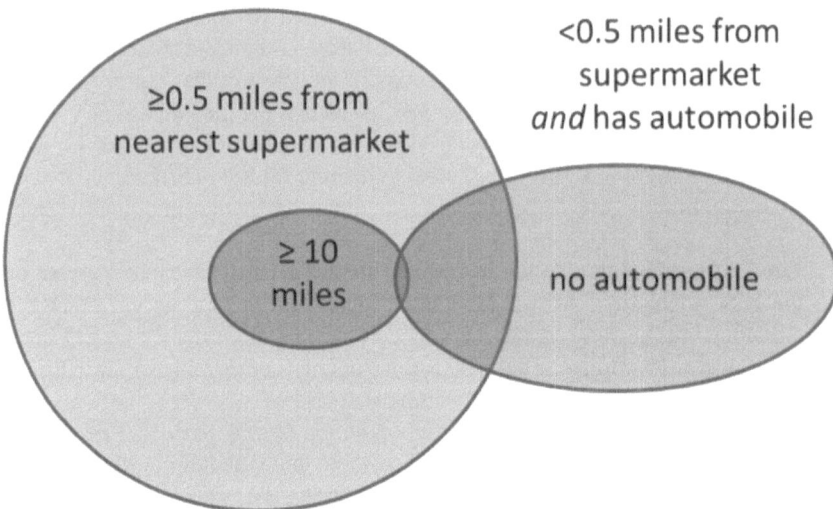

Figure 3.1   A concept of inadequate food retail access at the household level
Note: The circle at left represents households located at least 0.5 miles from a supermarket. A subset of these households are located at least 10 miles from a supermarket. The oval at right represents households with no vehicle. Darker shading in the intersection represents inadequate food retail access.

is 0.5 miles or 1 mile for people who lack a vehicle and a longer distance for people who have a vehicle. As an illustrative example (see Figure 3.1), one could say a household has inadequate access if (a) it lacks a vehicle and lives more than 0.5 miles from the nearest supermarket or (b) it has a vehicle and lives more than 10 miles from the nearest supermarket. This framework easily may be adapted for other threshold distances, such as 1 mile for households that lack a vehicle.

Data and methods

This study used geographic information for all census block groups within 50 primary sampling units (PSUs), which were counties or groups of counties in 27 states. The PSUs were drawn by Mathematica Policy Research, Inc., as the first stage of sampling for USDA's Food Acquisition and Purchase Survey (FoodAPS), a new national food expenditure survey (Kirlin and Denbaly 2013). Within the PSUs, the FoodAPS survey sampled approximately 5,000 households in 400 secondary sampling units (SSUs). None of the FoodAPS household data or SSU identifiers were used in this study, which only needed geographic-level data from the 50 PSUs.

The sample size was 33,604 block groups (after excluding 3 block groups that had implausibly high population densities, which we attributed to incorrect land area estimates). The analysis block groups belonged to 11,747 census tracts in 91 counties in the 50 PSUs. The block-group analysis file included two types of variables: (a) variables that were originally acquired at the block-group level (such as Census Bureau demographic characteristics for block groups), and (b) variables that describe the retail environment at varying distances from the population-weighted centroid of the block group.

This study used the same 2010 retailer location data that USDA/ERS used in FARA, combining information from TDLinx and USDA/FNS Store Tracking and Redemption System (STARS). Nielsen TDLinx is a commercial database of retailers selling consumer packaged goods, including food. FNS uses STARS to monitor and manage retailers authorized to participate in the federal government's Supplemental Assistance Nutrition Program (SNAP), formerly known as food stamps. Our analysis is based on counts of retailers located within a specified distance from the population-weighted block-group centroid. FARA, by contrast, is based on 0.5-km square grids rather than concentric circles. In FARA, the entire country was divided into 0.5-km square grids and then population data was allocated to these grids. The distance to the nearest supermarket was measured for each grid cell by calculating the distance between the geographic center of the 0.5-km square grid that contains estimates of the population and the center of the grid with the nearest supermarket. This study used block groups rather than 0.5-km square grids, because we lacked access to 0.5-km grid data, and block groups were judged to be adequately disaggregated.

At the block-group level, this study made no assumption that residents shopped within the block group itself. Instead, they were assumed to shop anywhere in the retail environment that surrounded the block-group centroid. We estimated counts for supermarkets and superstores at linear distances of 0.5 miles, 1 mile, 5 miles, 10 miles, and 20 miles from the population-weighted centroid of the block group. The commonly-used conventions (such as a 0.5-mile or 1-mile radius in urban areas or a 10-mile radius in rural areas) are special cases that can be analyzed using this data source.

For clarity, in the initial analysis of underlying relationships across block-group variables, this study used an absolute poverty standard for defining high-poverty areas. A high-poverty block group was defined as one with ≥ 20 percent of the population in poverty. The analysis used 4 population density levels, ranked from least to most dense: low, 0–1k persons per square mile; medium, 1k–5k persons per square mile; high, 5k–10k persons per square mile; very high, 10k+ persons per square mile. We removed from the analysis 3 outlier block groups with implausible population density greater than 300,000 persons per square mile (a density much greater than that of Manhattan). Block groups in rural census tracts are predominantly in density level 1. Block groups in urban census tracts are more numerous, and they are split evenly between density levels 2, 3, and 4.

The first four sections of the analysis address the four empirical questions noted in the introduction, describing the relationships among variables related to food access at the block-group level. The final section of analysis discusses issues of aggregation from a detailed geographic level (block group) to a broader geographic level (census tract).

Results

Poverty and proximity to supermarkets

First, consider the relationship between poverty and proximity to supermarkets. Overall, 26.1 percent of block groups were high-poverty, and these block groups contained 25.4 percent of the population. Because census block groups by design have roughly similar population sizes, weighting block groups by population made only small differences to the empirical results, so this study reports unweighted counts of block groups. High-poverty block groups (one quarter of all block groups) contained 60.6 percent of poor people. Lower-poverty block groups (three quarters of all block groups) contained the remaining 39.4 percent of poor people.

Fewer than 1 out of each 2,000 block groups (0.03 percent) lacked a supermarket within 20 miles, and another 1 out of 300 block groups (0.32 percent) lacked a supermarket within 10 miles (Table 3.1). At the other end of the spectrum, 43.9 percent of block groups had a supermarket within 0.5 miles, and another 35.2 percent of block groups had a supermarket between 0.5 miles and 1 mile away. In between the two extremes, 20.6 percent of block groups had a nearest supermarket between 1 and 10 miles away.

The high-poverty block groups had better access to supermarkets than other block groups did, on average. 85.6 percent of high-poverty block groups had a supermarket within 1 mile. By contrast, only 76.8 percent of lower-poverty block groups had a supermarket within this distance. Thus, most block groups had fairly good proximity to a nearest supermarket. Surprisingly, low-income block groups on average had better proximity than high-income block groups did.

Population density and proximity to supermarkets

Second, consider the relationship between population density and proximity to the nearest supermarket. Among block groups in the lowest-density level, only 6.1 percent are within 0.5 miles of a supermarket and another 15.8 percent are between 0.5 and 1 miles of a supermarket (Table 3.2). By contrast, among block groups in the highest-density level, 72.5 percent are within 0.5 miles of a supermarket.

Table 3.1 Frequency of having a nearest supermarket at each distance (in miles) for block groups with and without a high poverty rate

Block group poverty	Distance to nearest supermarket (in miles)					
	0 to 0.5	*0.5 to 1*	*1 to 10*	*10 to 20*	*>20*	*Total*
	# Block groups (row %)					
Not high poverty	10,029	8,968	5,659	88	6	24,750
	(40.52)	(36.23)	(22.86)	(0.36)	(0.02)	(100.00)
High poverty	4,655	2,817	1,230	18	5	8,725
	(53.35)	(32.29)	(14.10)	(0.21)	(0.06)	(100.00)
Total	14,684	11,785	6,889	106	11	33,475
	(43.87)	(35.21)	(20.58)	(0.32)	(0.03)	(100.00)

Note: High-poverty block groups have a poverty rate greater than or equal to 20%.

Table 3.2 Frequency of having a nearest supermarket at each distance (in miles) at each of four population density levels

Population density	Distance to nearest supermarket (in miles)					
	0 to 0.5	*0.5 to 1*	*1 to 10*	*10 to 20*	*>20*	*Total*
	# Block groups (row %)					
Low	229 (6.09)	592 (15.75)	2,821 (75.05)	106 (2.82)	11 (0.29)	3,759 (100.00)
Medium	2,567 (26.30)	4,388 (44.95)	2,805 (28.74)	1 (0.01)	0 (0.00)	9.761 (100.00)
High	4,408 (45.49)	4,255 (43.92)	1,026 (10.59)	0 (0.00)	0 (0.00)	9689 (100.00)
Very high	7,495 (72.53)	2,570 (24.87)	268 (2.59)	0 (0.00)	0 (0.00)	10,333 (100.00)
Total	14,699 (43.82)	11,805 (35.19)	6,920 (20.63)	107 (0.32)	11 (0.03)	33,542 (100.00)

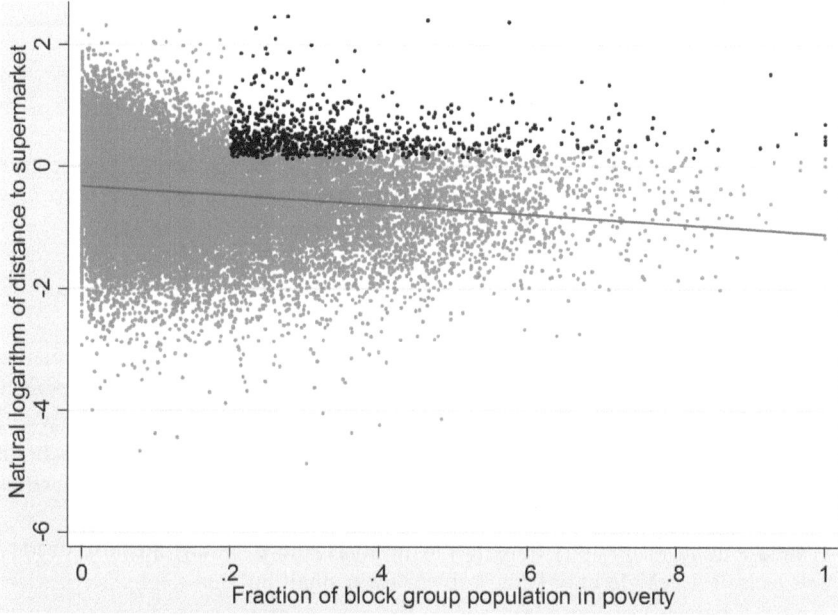

Figure 3.2   The natural logarithm of distance to the nearest supermarket, as a function of the poverty rate, in urban areas

Note: black color indicates the poverty rate is high (greater than 20%) and the nearest supermarket is 1 mile away or farther; the vertical axis shows the natural logarithm of the distance to the nearest supermarket in miles (the logarithmic scale is used for display, because the dependent variable is highly right-skewed).

For urban areas, Figure 3.2 shows block-group poverty rates on the horizontal axis and the natural logarithm of block-group miles to the nearest supermarket, ln(distance), on the vertical axis. Block groups farther than a mile from a supermarket have ln(distance) greater than zero. In the figure, there is not much correlation between ln(distance) and the poverty rate, and what little correlation exists is negative. The block groups that are both high-poverty and greater than one mile from the nearest supermarket are in the top right quadrant, marked in black.

This figure shows that definitional thresholds strongly influence descriptions of supermarket access that are based on distance and poverty rates. The block groups marked in black are not a standalone cluster in this two-dimensional space. On the contrary, an analyst using a distance threshold slightly different than one mile, or a poverty rate threshold slightly different than 20 percent, would have generated a much different estimate of the fraction of block groups that suffers from poor supermarket access. Moreover, the block groups illustrated in black are overshadowed by the larger number of block groups in the top left and bottom right quadrants. The block groups in the top left quadrant have poverty rates below 20 percent, but they are far from the nearest supermarket and they include large numbers of poor people (we noted earlier that almost two fifths of poor people live in block groups with poverty rates below 20 percent). The block groups in the bottom right quadrant have exceptionally high rates of poverty, and they may face serious problems with the quality of the food environment, but they do enjoy close proximity to the nearest supermarket.

Thus, much more than poverty, population density was a powerful predictor of proximity to a nearest supermarket. Nearly all block groups with very high population density had a nearest supermarket no more than 1 mile away.

Vehicle access and proximity to supermarkets

Third, consider the relationship between vehicle availability and supermarket access. In block groups with a supermarket less than 0.5 miles away, 15.3 percent of households lacked a vehicle (Table 3.3). For in-between block groups, with a nearest supermarket between 1 and 10 miles away, 4.7 percent of households lacked a vehicle. In block groups with a nearest supermarket between 10 and 20 miles away, 4.6 percent of households lacked a vehicle.

Thus, vehicle availability is highest in the areas where vehicles are most needed. Yet, lack of a vehicle may be a problem for a small but non-negligible fraction (almost 5 percent) of those households that are at least 1 mile from the nearest supermarket.

Table 3.3 Percentage of households having no vehicle, for block groups with nearest supermarket in each distance category

	Distance to nearest supermarket (in miles)				
	0 to 0.5	*0.5 to 1*	*1 to 10*	*10 to 20*	*>20*
Mean % with no vehicle	15.34	8.04	4.71	4.55	5.71

Proximity to supermarkets based on area characteristics

Fourth, consider the proximity to supermarkets in block groups with particular levels of population density and vehicle access. This fourth empirical question helps us to understand relative distance methods, such as TRF's approach to identifying LSAs, which was described in the background section.

This study's relative distance analysis, loosely motivated by TRF's approach, used the same 4 population density levels as in our earlier results. We defined a block group as "high vehicle" if the rate of vehicle access was greater than 80 percent, and "low vehicle" otherwise. We stratified all block groups into low-income (having a high poverty rate or low relative income or both) and not-low-income categories. TRF uses only higher-income areas (defined as having median income above 120 percent of the poverty guideline) to establish adequate benchmark distances.

In our analysis, as in TRF (2011), the low-density block groups had high vehicle access rates (Table 3.4). The mean distance to the nearest supermarket among these predominantly low-density block groups was about 4 miles (4.18 miles in low-income block groups and 3.93 miles in other block groups). By contrast, for block groups with the highest population density level, the mean distance to the nearest supermarket was much smaller, ranging from 0.37 to 0.57 miles depending on vehicle access and low-income status. These benchmark distances are similar to the results TRF (2011) found for high-density areas.

Thus, although our relative distance approach did not seek exactly to replicate the TRF approach, we observed the same patterns that TRF observed. High-vehicle high-population-density areas tend to have short benchmark distances of much less than 1 mile, which means that such block groups generally are within 1 mile of a supermarket.

Table 3.4 Benchmark distances for several population density and vehicle access categories

Population density	Mean distance in miles (% of all block groups)			
	Not lower income		Lower income	
	High Vehicle	Low Vehicle	High Vehicle	Low Vehicle
1 (lowest density)	3.93	—	4.18	—
	(13.0)		(7.5)	
2	1.13	—	0.97	0.87
	(35.4)		(15.7)	(4.6)
3	0.76	—	0.75	0.71
	(30.3)		(19.8)	(6.3)
4 (highest density)	0.57	0.37	0.57	0.42
	(15.4)	(4.3)	(25.1)	(20.1)

Note: Empty cells indicate that few people live in areas with that combination of population density and vehicle access.

Aggregating to the census tract

In urban areas, a block group generally is sufficiently small that the population-weighted centroid can be treated as the location where people live. We recognize that rural block groups are larger, but, in this study, we nonetheless use the population-weighted block group centroid as an approximation of the location where residents live. In yet larger geographic units such as census tracts, one always must recognize that the food environment is different for residents of different neighborhoods within the unit. Building on the basic block-group level results in the previous section, we next investigate issues of aggregating to the census-tract level in the low-income low-access approach. Some of the lessons from this analysis may apply to other approaches as well.

USDA's FARA identifies census tracts that are both (1) a low-income tract and (2) a low-access tract (meaning that the households have poor proximity to the nearest supermarket). It is comparatively straightforward to define a low-income census tract, using the same approach as was used previously to define a low-income block group. Low income, in FARA, means having a poverty rate of at least 20 percent (as in the previous section) or having low median income relative to other parts of the same metropolitan area or state. While the previous section showed that 26 percent of block groups had high poverty, 42.2 percent of census tracts qualify as low-income using this more expansive definition (Table 3.5).

It is more difficult to define low access at the census-tract level than at the block-group level. The issue is that supermarket access is an attribute of a very specific geographic location, such as a block-group centroid (in the previous section) or a small 0.5-km square grid cell (in USDA's FARA estimates). In contrast with a block group, a census tract is too large an area for the distance from the census-tract centroid to be a useful concept. Hence, FARA based its tract-level definition of low-access on a particular aggregation: a low-access census tract is one in which at least 500 people reside in low-access grid cells, or 33 percent of the tract population resides in low-access grid cells, or both. While the previous section showed that 20.9 percent of block groups had no supermarket within 1 mile, this census-tract analysis found that 25.5 percent of census tracts qualify as low access using this approach (Table 3.5). It is common to have low-access census tracts that include some neighborhoods with adequate food retail access.

Overall, 879 out of 11,735 census tracts (or 7.5 percent of all census tracts) met both the low-access *and* low-income criteria. Low-income census tracts are less likely than other census tracts to be classified as low-access tracts. Of those census tracts classified as having low income, 17.8 percent also had low access. Of census tracts that were not low-income, 31.1 percent had low access (Table 3.5). To summarize, the census-tract level analysis was more likely than the earlier block-group level analysis to classify a geographical area as an area with inadequate food retail. Yet, the basic relationship between income status and food retail access status remained the same. Low-income census tracts have comparatively good access to supermarkets.

Table 3.5 Joint frequency for census tracts having low income and low access

Income status	Access status		
	Not low	*Low*	*Total*
		# Census Tracts (row %)	
Not low income	4,672 (68.88)	2,111 (31.12)	6,783 (100.00)
Low income	4,073 (82.25)	879 (17.75)	4,952 (100.00)
Total	8,745 (74.52)	2,990 (25.48)	11,735 (100.00)

Note: The ERS Food Access Research Atlas (FARA) classifies a tract with both low income and low access as a "food desert."

Discussion

There is substantial policy interest in classifying geographic areas according to the adequacy of the local food retail environment and in measuring the prevalence of poor access conditions. Three leading approaches share some similarities in methods and motivation, but they differ in key respects and lead to substantially different conclusions about food retail adequacy.

The approaches studied here each measure the distance to the nearest supermarket and compare it to a threshold distance thought to indicate an acceptable burden for grocery shopping. In the low-income low-access approach, USDA Economic Research Service (2009) used time-based measures for walking and driving to develop estimates of walkable and drivable distances. For walking, the authors assumed a walking speed of 2 miles per hour and a 15-minute walking time to arrive at a 0.5 mile radius for "high" access (in urban areas). Others (Algert, Agrawal, and Lewis 2006; Apparicio, Cloutier, and Shearmur 2007; California Center for Public Health Advocacy, PolicyLink, and UCLA Center for Health Policy Research 2008) have used similar definitions of walkability. For driving, USDA's Economic Research Service assumed a driving speed of 40 miles per hour and a 15-minute drive to arrive at a 10-mile radius for "high" access in rural areas. Clearly, if one uses a smaller threshold distance, one is systematically more likely to classify a particular location as having inadequate food retail conditions. Conversely, if one uses a larger threshold distance, one finds fewer such areas. Hence, a lot depends on the choice of threshold distance. The findings show that the choice of the threshold point could make a sizable difference in the number of locations that are designated as limited access.

Each approach implicitly sought to take account of the fact that a reasonable threshold distance may be different for households with and without vehicles, but the methods for taking account of vehicle availability differed considerably. If the population of concern is people who live further than a threshold distance and lack a vehicle, then FARA's vehicle-based measure seems to be the most direct approach.

Using low-income status at the census-tract level has some shortcomings as a method for identifying this population. Because low-income areas are more likely than other areas to have a supermarket nearby, the low-income low-access approach actually excludes many areas that are not low-income, but which have particularly long distances to the nearest supermarket. Recall from the first section of results that almost 40 percent of poor people live in neighborhoods that are not high-poverty neighborhoods. One could argue that the low-income low-access approach excludes one of the most commonly deprived populations, which is poor people in non-poor neighborhoods that lack a supermarket.

Similarly, the relative distance approach would be an indirect way of identifying areas where people lack a vehicle and live too far from a supermarket. In some areas with large threshold distances, it seems possible that households without a vehicle would face great hardship. In other areas, a threshold distance of less than 0.5 miles may be too short. In such areas, many residents without vehicles may be classified as having limited supermarket access even if they are well-satisfied with nearby supermarkets at distances of between 0.5 miles and 1 mile.

We conclude that neither the low-income low-access approach nor the relative distance approach serves well as a method for accounting for vehicle access, but we recognize that there may be other motivations for these approaches. It could be that low income is not intended as a proxy for low vehicle availability, but instead there is a more direct reason why people in low-income neighborhoods without a supermarket should be at greater disadvantage than people in other neighborhoods without a supermarket. For example, community development in low-income neighborhoods could be the policy goal. Likewise, there could be a more direct motivation for the relative distance approach, such as concerns over equity of access.

Our results suggest some recommendations for future work in measuring food retail adequacy. First, it is good to state explicitly the household-level or individual-level condition that represents inadequate food retail access. For example, the underlying household-level condition might be one of the three conditions studied in this study: (1) poverty plus lack of a nearby supermarket, or (2) lack of a vehicle plus lack of a nearby supermarket, or (3) lack of a supermarket as close as one typically expects in neighborhoods with similar population density. Alternatively, the household-level condition might address issues beyond those covered here, such as lack of fresh fruits and vegetables at a particular price point. Second, when it is necessary to aggregate from granular geographic data to larger areas such as census tracts or counties, it is good to do so in a fashion that preserves the underlying information about the extent of hardship. Current methods of aggregation may cautiously classify some census tracts as having inadequate access even if many block groups or smaller geographic units contained in the census tracts have adequate food retail access.

The research literature on food retail adequacy may have policy implications. In particular, policy-makers may choose to target areas for subsidies or tax incentives to attract additional commercial supermarkets, or they may use zoning rules to guide retailer location decisions. When research on food retail adequacy is used in this fashion, it is especially important that the choice of threshold distance and assumptions about vehicle adequacy match actual consumer behavior. For example, if one assumed that low-income households in a particular community seek to shop for groceries within a 0.5-mile radius, when in fact vehicle availability rates are high and households in this community usually patronize lower-priced retailers at greater distances, then it could be a substantial policy error to subsidize the introduction of a new supermarket. To determine locations where market outcomes have been unsatisfactory and where a new supermarket may be encouraged, it is good first to recognize and assess population density, vehicle availability, and the proximity of other supermarkets.

Notes

1 This chapter is modified from an article originally published by IFAMA, and is included in this volume with permission: Wilde, P., J. Llobrera, and M. Ver Ploeg. 2014. "Population Density, Poverty, and Food Retail Access in the United States: An Empirical Approach." *International Food and Agribusiness Management Review* 17(A): 171–186. Archived at: www.ifama.org.
2 This work is the responsibility of the authors and is not attributable to Tufts University, Insight Policy Research, or the USDA.

References

Algert, S.J., Agrawal, A., and Lewis, D.S. 2006. Disparities in access to fresh produce in low-income neighborhoods in Los Angeles. *American Journal of Preventive Medicine* 30 (5): 365–370.

Apparicio, P., Cloutier, M.S., and Shearmur, R. 2007. The case of Montreal's missing food deserts: Evaluation of accessibility to food supermarkets. *International Journal of Health Geographies* 6 (4).

Benson, B.L., and Faminow, M.D. 1985. An alternative view of pricing in retail food markets. *American Journal of Agricultural Economics* 67 (2): 296–306.

Bitler, M., and Haider, S.J. 2011. An economic view of food deserts in the United States. *Journal of Policy Analysis and Management* 30 (1): 153–176.

Bonanno, A., and Lopez, R.A. 2009. Competition effects of supermarket services. *American Journal of Agricultural Economics* 91 (3): 555–568.

Broda, C., Leibtag, E., and Weinstein, D.E. 2009. The role of prices in measuring the poor's living standards. *The Journal of Economic Perspectives* 23 (2): 77–97.

California Center for Public Health Advocacy, PolicyLink, and UCLA Center for Health Policy Research. 2008. *Designed for Disease: The Link between Local Food Environments and Obesity and Diabetes*.

Chen, S., Florax, R.J.G.M., and Snyder, S.D. 2010. Does where you live make you fat? Obesity and access to chain grocers. *Economic Geography* 86: 431–452.

Cole, N. 1997. *Evaluation of the Expanded EBT Demonstration in Maryland: Patterns of Food Stamp and Cash Welfare Benefit Redemption.* Report submitted to U.S. Department of Agriculture, Food and Nutrition Service, by Abt Associates, Inc.

Cotterill, R.W. 1986. Market power in the retail food industry: Evidence from Vermont. *The Review of Economics and Statistics* 68 (3): 379–386.

Economic Research Service (ERS). 2013. U.S. Department of Agriculture (USDA). Food Access Research Atlas (FARA). Available online at www.ers.usda.gov/data-products/food-access-research-atlas.aspx (accessed August 2, 2013).

Fik, T.J. 1988. Spatial competition and price reporting in retail food markets. *Economic Geography* 64 (4): 29–44.

Gibson, D.M. 2011. The neighborhood food environment and adult weight status: Estimates from longitudinal data. *American Journal of Public Health* 101: 71–78.

Gittelsohn, J., and Lee, K. 2013. Integrating educational, environmental, and behavioral economic strategies may improve the effectiveness of obesity interventions. *Applied Economic Perspectives and Policy* 35 (1): 52–68.

Gittelsohn, J., Rowan, M., and Gadhoke, P. 2012. Interventions in small food stores to change the food environment, improve diet, and reduce risk of chronic disease. *Preventing Chronic Disease* 9: E59.

Huff, D.L. 1964. Defining and estimating a trading area. *The Journal of Marketing* 28: 34–38.

Kirlin, J.A., and Denbaly, M. 2013. FoodAPS National Household Food Acquisition and Purchase Survey, U.S. Department of Agriculture, Economic Research Service, July 2013. Available online at www.ers.usda.gov/data-products/foodaps-national-household-food-acquisition-and-purchase-survey.aspx (accessed August 2, 2013).

Leung, C.W., Laraia, B.A., Kelly, M., Nickleach, D., Adler, N.E., Kushi, L.H., and Yen, I.H. 2011. The influence of neighborhood food stores on change in young girls' body mass index. *American Journal of Preventive Medicine* 41: 43–51.

Rose, D. 2010. Access to healthy food: A key focus for research on domestic food insecurity. *Journal of Nutrition* 140: 1167–1169.

The Reinvestment Fund (TRF). 2011. *Limited Supermarket Access Analysis: Summary of TRF's Methodology*. Available online at www.trfund.com/resource/downloads/policypubs/LSAMethodology2011.pdf (accessed May 24, 2016).

U.S. Census Bureau. 2010 Terms and Concepts. Available online at www.census.gov/geo/reference/terms.html (accessed May 24, 2016).

USDA Economic Research Service. 2009. *Access to Affordable and Nutritious Food – Measuring and Understanding Food Deserts and Their Consequences: Report to Congress*. Contributors: Ver Ploeg, M., Breneman, V., Farrigan, T., Hamrick, K., Hopkins, D., Kaufman, P., Lin, B.H., Nord, M., Smith, T.A., Williams, R., Kinnison, R., Olander, C., Singh, A., and Tuckermanty, E. Washington, DC: U.S. Department of Agriculture, Economic Research Service.

USDA Economic Research Service. 2012. *Access to Affordable and Nutritious Food: Updated Estimates of Distance to Economic Supermarkets Using 2010 Data*. Contributors: Ver Ploeg, M., Breneman, V., Dutko, P., Williams, R., Snyder, S., Dicken, C., and Kaufman, P. Washington, DC: U.S. Department of Agriculture, Economic Research Service.

4 Super-sized strategies for improved health

Does reducing the density of fast food restaurants matter?

Bakeyah Nelson and Karen Banks

The consumption of fast food has soared as fast food establishments have become ubiquitous throughout the American landscape (Freeman 2007). There is no standard definition of fast food, so we define it as food that is pre-made and prepared for quick consumption, ordered or served over a counter or at a drive-through window, and paid for before consumption. Since the 1970s, the number of fast food restaurants and the amount of food consumed away from home has increased at an exceptional rate. In 2012, 43.1 percent of all meals were eaten away from home as compared to just 25.9 percent in 1970, a 66 percent increase.

This increase in the access to and consumption of food away from home has resulted in the fast food industry being labeled a main contributor to the current obesity epidemic. Similar to the increases in consumption in food away from home, the obesity rate has more than doubled since the early 1970s, when 14 percent of adults were classified as medically obese (Cutler, Glaeser, and Shapiro 2003) to over 30 percent of adults considered obese in 2012 (Ogden et al. 2014). Some social groups experience even higher rates of obesity. While in general the disparity in obesity rates along racial/ethnic and socioeconomic lines has narrowed over time, African Americans, Hispanics and individuals of lower-incomes experience higher obesity rates than non-Hispanic Whites (Hu 2008). These trends, in part, are assumed to be a result of less access to healthy food options and greater reliance on cheap, energy dense food that can be purchased at fast food outlets (Binkley et al., 2000; Prentice and Jebb, 2003; Duffey et al., 2007; Duffey and Popkin, 2011), which are more prevalent in communities of color and low-income areas (Block et al., 2004). Consequently, the public health community has responded by promoting efforts to limit the availability of fast food as one approach to combat obesity, among other objectives (Sturm and Cohen, 2009).

The Centers for Disease Control and Prevention (CDC) and other public health stakeholders have put forth policy strategies to change the built environment to promote healthier lifestyle choices and limit unhealthy options, including restricting the density of fast food outlets through zoning. This strategy rests on a basic causal argument: 1) closer proximity to fast food outlets results in higher consumption of fast food, 2) higher consumption of fast food leads to weight gain, and 3) the resulting weight gain from consuming fast food is bad for one's health and leads to obesity and obesity-related diseases, such as diabetes, hypertension, and heart disease. A great deal of research has gone into understanding the relationship between these assumptions, with so far mixed results that point to an association only in certain instances (Fleischhacker et al. 2011; Fraser et al. 2010; Rosenheck 2008). As such, it is unclear to what extent a ban on fast food outlets, by way of zoning, will have on reducing and preventing obesity.

An overview of the evidence about the relationship between fast food access, consumption and obesity is presented here in an effort to challenge the prevailing view that limiting the density of fast food restaurants through zoning is an effective strategy for obesity prevention. We examine the relevant literature on the relationship between 1) the density of fast food outlets and obesity, 2) the proximity of fast food outlets and consumption, and 3) the consumption of fast food and weight. While this review is not intended as an exhaustive assessment of all literature, all relevant systematic reviews of the literature on this topic conducted by other researchers are included. Ultimately, we conclude that zoning restrictions on fast food outlets are likely to have minimal impact on obesity. Therefore, we ask: to what extent is the investment to pass local control measures to limit the commercial development of fast food outlets an effective use of time, resources, and political will? Additionally, to what extent does this strategy perpetuate socioeconomically stratified communities? We then propose alternative policy strategies that may be more effective and perhaps should be prioritized to increase the consumption of healthy food and reduce fast food consumption patterns among communities of color and low-income.

A brief history of zoning and public health

There is growing evidence that the built environment can influence health behaviors known to prevent chronic diseases, such as eating a nutritious diet and engaging in physical activity (CDC 2011). Zoning, a public policy tool used to regulate land use, has a direct impact on a community's built environment – the man-made features within a community and the design of those features – and a troublesome history in the U.S., particularly as it impacts minority communities. The legal authority to zone land is granted to states through the Tenth Amendment by way of state police powers that can be used for the purpose of protecting the health, safety and welfare of the public (Nolan and Salkin 2007). Intended to keep "incompatible" land uses apart, zoning has historically been used to address public health challenges such as reducing exposure to hazardous air pollutants and minimizing the spread of infectious diseases (Coburn 2009). While zoning has successfully served to protect public health, for the most part it has also served to segregate social groups and, in part because low-income populations also tend to be clustered near highways, factories, and other pollution producing facilities, has led to disparities in health outcomes such as higher rates of respiratory illnesses, hypertension, heart disease, and cancer, among others (Rossen and Pollack 2012).

Exclusionary zoning practices that dictated minimum lot sizes and housing types served to exclude low-income and minority groups from certain neighborhoods and to preserve the property values of predominantly wealthy communities (Silver 1997; Coburn 2009). Zoning was used to enforce racial segregation (Silver 1997), a practice that has had lingering, negative impacts on the landscape of African American communities (Kwate 2008). Residential segregation is considered a major contributor to disparities in health outcomes by way of differences in the distribution of resources across neighborhoods, and the concentration of poverty in only certain neighborhoods (Acevedo-Garcia and Lochner 2003). For example, Kwate (2008) asserts that racial residential segregation has led to the over concentration of fast food outlets in African American communities.

Moreover, studies have documented differences in the distribution of resources across communities. Toxic waste dumps and other environmental hazards (Landrine and Corral 2009), opportunities for physical activity (Active Living Research, 2011), and the availability of both healthy and unhealthy food resources (Neckerman et al. 2009; Kwate et al. 2009) are inequitably distributed across neighborhoods. Thus, it has been argued that, along with the concentration of poverty, the inequitable distribution of resources for healthy lifestyle choices across neighborhoods is one factor fueling poor health outcomes experienced in low-income communities, which in urban America tend to be heavily populated by racial minorities (Kwate 2008; Neckerman et al. 2009; Rossen and Pollack 2012). Kwate (2008) demonstrated that these communities have significantly higher access to fast food outlets in their neighborhoods relative to more affluent, White areas. Such history explains current efforts to encourage healthy lifestyle choices by using zoning for public welfare to limit the density of "unhealthy" fast food outlets. This strategy however, has the potential to repeat history by inadvertently leading to further disenfranchisement in low-income areas and communities of color.

Fast food availability and obesity

It is uncertain whether efforts to limit access to fast food, by way of zoning, will lead to a significant reduction in obesity. Given the negative history between zoning and public health in communities of color and neighborhoods of low-income it is critical to scrutinize the potential unintended consequences of regulatory controls to change the food environment. To better examine the extent to which the evidence supports regulating access to fast food, we applied criteria developed by Austin Bradford Hill and used by epidemiologists to explore causality between an exposure and a health outcome. While these criteria are often applied implicitly to evaluate epidemiological studies, we explicitly apply them to highlight their relevance in efforts to evaluate available evidence that may be used to inform the development of public policies to address public health challenges. It is important to note however, that disease causation is complex and, with the exception of the temporality criterion, not meeting any of Hill's criteria does not necessarily dismiss a causal relationship (Rothman, Greenland, and Lash 2008). Table 4.1 (below) presents the Hill criteria along with the studies reviewed and their findings. We then discuss the potential impacts of limiting fast food

Table 4.1 Bradford Hill criteria of causality and their relation to a sample of studies examining the relationship between fast-food availability, consumption and obesity

Hill criteria	Author(s)/year	Relationship (+/-)
Strength of Association - Stronger associations are more likely to reflect true causal relationships between an exposure and a hazard and less likely to be a result of chance, bias or confounding variables (Remington, Brownson & Wegner, 2010). While many studies show a positive association, the associations have been very weak.	Maddock 2006	In a state-level model that explains 70 percent of obesity across states, fast food outlets accounted for only 6 percent of the state-level variation in obesity rates. (+)
	Currie et al. 2010	A positive association was found between the supply in fast food and obesity among ninth graders and pregnant women – particularly, African American women. A 0.5 percent increase in obesity over the past 30 years and a 2.7 percent increase in obesity over the past 10 years were observed. (+)
	Boone-Heinonen et al. 2011	Among low-income men, fast-food consumption increases by 0.34 percent when fast food outlets are within 1 - 3 km of a home. (+)
	Forsyth et al. 2012	Among adolescent males, the more fast food outlets there are within 1600 m of one's home or school, the more frequently a young male will consume fast food. (+) Among low-income men, a one percent increase in the availability of fast food within 1 km of a home is related to a 0.13 percent increase in the consumption of fast food. (+)
Consistency - considers whether results are consistent when using diverse research designs, study populations, geographic areas, and time (Remington, Brownson & Wegner, 2010). While many studies have shown a positive association, the findings have been inconsistent across varying populations and places.	Fraser et al. 2010	Six out of the 12 studies reviewed by Fraser found an association between fast food availability and obesity while seven studies found negative or no association.
	Fleischhacker et al. 2011	Seven out of 15 studies reviewed found an association between fast food availability and obesity while eight studies did not find a relationship. (-)
	Dunn et al. 2012	Increasing availability of fast food increases fast food consumption among Black but not White rural residents. However, the authors concluded that the results may stem from differences in the socioeconomic characteristics between these groups. (+)

Temporality – refers to whether an exposure occurred prior to the onset of a disease or health outcome (Remington, Brownson & Wegner, 2010). Temporality is considered the only "absolute" criterion for establishing causality. Note that in order to establish a causal relationship in this case, the consumption of fast food, along with the development of obesity would have to increase as a result of an increasing supply of fast food outlets in a defined geographic area.	Pereira et al. 2005	This study found a positive association between frequency of fast food consumption and weight gain over a 15-year period. However, this study captured consumption but did not address access to fast food. (+)
	Currie et al. 2010	This study controlled for current proximity to fast food outlets and examined the effect of an increasing supply of fast food establishments on weight gain. The authors demonstrated among certain groups, when the supply of fast food increases there are corresponding incremental weight increases. However, it is concluded that efforts to limit the availability of fast food outlets in residential areas will not have a considerable impact on obesity among individuals with transportation options although there maybe some benefit around schools and inner city neighborhoods. (+)
	Boone-Heinonen et al. 2011	Greater fast food access was positively associated with higher fast food consumption and the magnitude of the relationship was most pronounced among low-income men. (+)
	Pereria et al. 2005 and Duffey et al. 2007	These studies demonstrated that consumption of fast food is associated with increased energy intake and higher BMI. (+)
	Fraser et al. 2010 and Fleischhacker et al. 2011	Reviews of the literature do not consistently show that fast food density is associated with obesity. (-)
Theoretical Plausibility/Coherence – considers whether there is a theoretical basis for an observed association and whether that association is coherent with other scientific knowledge (Remington, Brownson & Wegner, 2010). We assert that it is conceivable that the more available a particular food choice, the more individuals will consume, within their cost constraints and taste preferences. However, many studies examining this issue have not considered other factors that influence daily eating behaviors. Furthermore, there is no clear indication that people who consume fast food are overweight or that people that live near fast food were not overweight prior to the proliferation of fast food establishments.		

Table 4.1 Continued

Hill criteria	Author(s)/year	Relationship (+/-)
Biological Gradient - refers to the extent to which the risk of disease increases with increasing exposure to a hazard – in this case fast food outlets (Remington, Brownson & Wegner, 2010). While these studies demonstrate a dose-response relationship between increasing fast food consumption and weight gain, it is unknown whether those individuals that consume fast food more frequently in these studies also live in closer proximity to fast food outlets or whether they engage in less physical activity than those reporting less fast food consumption. With the exception of Pereira et al. (2005), most studies have not adjusted for physical activity, a potential confounder that significantly influences weight status (Fraser et al., 2010).	French et al. 2001

Bowman and Vinyard 2004 and Duffey et al. 2007 | Examined the relationship between the frequency of fast food consumption and weight status among women enrolled in a weight gain prevention intervention trial. Results indicated that over a 3-year period, increasing frequency of fast food consumption was found to be associated with higher energy and fat intake along with greater body weight. (+)

Both studies found individuals reporting consuming fast food had higher weight than those reporting less frequent consumption. (+) |

outlets in communities of color and low-income and discuss alternative strategies that may be more effective in curbing obesity.

For the most part, the results of the evaluation of the literature applying Hill's criteria for causality show a positive yet weak relationship between fast food availability, consumption and obesity. However, not all of the results were positive. It is important to note that there are inherent shortcomings with observational epidemiologic studies that result from systematic errors (bias) in their design (Ahern, Brown and Dukas, 2011; Richardson et al., 2011). One such shortcoming that bears relevance to this examination of the evidence is confounding, a bias that can distort the ostensible association between an exposure and an outcome by way of a third variable that also influences the outcome under study (Hu 2008). For example, physical activity is a potential confounder in fast food consumption and obesity-related studies. The magnitude of an association found between fast food intake and obesity is likely weaker when adjusting for physical activity. Yet most studies on fast food intake and obesity do not take physical activity into consideration (Peireira et al. 2005). While we too did not consider physical activity in our examination of the relationship between fast food availability and obesity, recognition of bias and confounding variables support our premise that this is a complex relationship, potentially influenced by multiple variables, including physical activity, individual and community-level socio-economic status, personal preference, and environmental factors.

Finally, in the most recent systematic review of over 60 studies in the literature, Cobb et al. (2015) assert that most studies on the impact of local food environments and obesity are methodologically weak and "associations between fast food outlet availability and obesity are predominantly null." The authors conclude that there is limited evidence supporting the association between local food environments and obesity (Cobb et al. 2015).

Case studies

The impact on obesity of zoning restrictions on fast food is still up for debate because, while a handful of cities have imposed zoning ordinances to limit the number of fast food outlets due to aesthetic or design concerns, so far only the City of Los Angeles has sought to ban fast food outlets based on public health concerns (Strum 2009).

Los Angeles, California

In 2008, the City of Los Angeles passed Ordinance No. 180130, an interim ordinance banning the development of new stand-alone fast food outlets in three areas of South Los Angeles. The interim ordinance was extended for two years, after which it expired but was replaced by an amendment to the City's General Plan that imposed six criteria on new stand-alone fast food establishments, including the requirement that new establishments be at least 0.5 miles from an existing fast food establishment (Bassford et al. 2012).

The rationale for the ordinance was an over-proliferation of fast food outlets in what is a predominantly lower-income area. This rationale – an inverse association between fast food availability and low-income or low socioeconomic status – is a consistent finding across the literature (Fleischhacker et al. 2011; Fraser et al. 2010; Forsyth et al. 2012; Hickson et al. 2011): the lower an area's average income, the more fast food outlets it contains. According to a story in the *Los Angeles Times*, South Los Angeles had a proportionally higher density of fast food outlets compared to the more affluent west side of the city; 45 percent of all restaurants in South Los Angeles were fast food restaurants compared to 16 percent in the west side of the city (Abdollah 2007).

The rationale for the ordinance prohibiting the development of new fast food outlets in South Los Angeles did not hold up in external evaluations. The density of fast food restaurants by population and in comparison to other types of restaurants in South Los Angeles was not significantly different, and was found to be even slightly less than other areas of Los Angeles (Strum 2009). One limitation of the ban was that it only applied to new stand-alone fast food restaurants, permitting the development of new establishments in existing retail centers and mixed-use developments. Community Health Councils, Inc. reported that a dozen new fast food restaurants opened under the interim ordinance. Additionally, the first study evaluating the effectiveness of the ban indicates that fast food consumption in South Los Angeles in fact *increased* since the ban, and finds no evidence that it has successfully reduced obesity (Sturm and Hattori 2015). Consistent with our evaluation of the literature through Hill's criteria for causality, the South Los Angeles ban on fast food outlets seems to fall short of the desired objective to protect public health.

Pasadena, Texas

According to local data from the Health of Houston Survey (2010), 66 percent of adults and 65 percent of children (age 12+) in the city of Pasadena, Texas, are overweight or obese. It is one of the highest rates of obesity within Harris County, which also is home to the much larger city of Houston. The fast food environment in Pasadena is similar to that of South Los Angeles, with approximately 42 percent of restaurants in the city being classified as fast food. Healthy Living Matters (HLM), a local initiative aimed at curbing childhood obesity in Harris County through policy and environmental change, developed a set of recommendations for the city to improve its food environment based on community input gathered through surveys, focus groups and interviews. While focus group participants cited the affordability and convenience of fast food as a barrier to healthy eating, the price of healthy food was the number one factor affecting their ability to eat healthy.

Restricting the development of additional fast food establishments was put forth as one policy strategy to address the obesity rate. However, Pasadena residents instead opted to enhance access to affordable, healthy food over restricting the availability of unhealthy food outlets. For example, one strategy implemented is to increase access to healthy options at schools and convenience stores in targeted zip codes. HLM partnered with the Pasadena Independent School District and the Houston-based nonprofit Brighter Bites to deliver fresh fruits and vegetables to families at selected elementary schools. Through this program, families receive weekly deliveries of fresh produce and children are also educated about how to choose healthier options. HLM also facilitated a partnership between CAN DO Houston and several other organizations and local corner stores to launch the Healthy Corner Store Network (HCSN) in Pasadena. At participating convenience stores, the initiative included increasing the availability of fresh produce, nutrition education and signage to promote healthier food options, healthy food demonstrations along with incentives, such as free produce giveaways to consumers who purchase healthy food options.

Another way the community is increasing access to healthy food is through a grant to launch a community-supported agriculture (CSA) campus in north Pasadena, one of the city's most socioeconomically disadvantaged areas. The CSA campus will enable residents to purchase shares of crops from an on-site farm in exchange for regular produce deliveries. In December 2015, Pasadena's City Council unanimously passed a Chapter 380 Economic Development Agreement with a vertical farming engineering company which granted the firm access to a vacant city building and tax incentives to establish what will become a farming, research, and education campus. In partnership with the local school district, health department, food bank and colleges, the campus will house a small scale indoor farm to grow for sale to residents and will offer educational and job training opportunities. The goal of the campus is to "train the next generation of farmers and provide a pipeline of skilled labor into the vertical farming industry" (Globe Newswire 2015). These community-driven initiatives are currently being implemented and have yet to be evaluated for their effectiveness in reducing obesity rates. However, in the event that these strategies are not effective at obesity reduction, at a minimum they create economic and educational opportunities for residents.

At the state level, legislation was proposed during the 84th Texas State Legislature that would have strengthened healthy food access in communities similar to Pasadena. House Bill 1485 (Rodrigues, Eddie et al.) would have established a grocery access investment fund to finance the construction, rehabilitation and/or expansion of grocery stores in low-income areas with limited supermarket access. However, the bill never got out of committee. As a result, for Texas residents, as for residents in most U.S. states for that matter, the onus of expanding access to healthy food – or limiting access to unhealthy food – remains primarily at the community level. While it is recognized that no one strategy will have an overwhelming influence on reducing obesity, in communities with limited time, resources and political capital, perhaps community-based strategies that strengthen educational and economic opportunities for low-income residents should be prioritized above those that limit them.

Discussion

Given the mixed and often weak association between fast food availability and obesity, to what extent is the investment to pass measures that restrict the development of fast food outlets an effective use of political capital, time, and resources? The relationship between the built environment, particularly the food environment, and public health is complex. It is compounded by individual preference (Forsyth et al. 2012; Gordon-Larsen 2014) and local contexts – social and cultural (Ford and Dzewaltowski 2008), and political and economic. What a person is able to buy – dictated by income and availability – and *wants* to buy – based on sensory appeal, marketing, familiarity, social influence, morals, and health – all influence what a person eats (Pollard, Kirk, and Cade 2002). What, then, are the indirect impacts on a community when fast food outlets are banned from the area? This question is especially pertinent in predominantly African American communities, which face higher proportions of concentrated poverty and residual effects from residential segregation policies that impacted the food landscape in these neighborhoods. Inappropriately applied policies, like zoning restrictions on fast food outlets, without appropriate support for improving the landscape could further disenfranchise already vulnerable populations.

Fast food, race, and community wellbeing

While the results of limiting fast food on public health are inconclusive, it is also yet to be understood, and examined, how banning fast food establishments will impact community wellbeing, particularly in low-income neighborhoods and predominantly African American communities. According to Wiseman and Brasher (2008), "community wellbeing is the combination of social, economic, environmental, cultural, and political conditions identified by individuals and their communities as essential for them to flourish and fulfill their potential." A consistent finding across the literature is an association between fast food availability and socioeconomic status with increased density of fast food outlets in low-income communities (Fleischhacker et al. 2011; Fraser et al. 2010; Forsyth et al. 2012; Hickson et al. 2011; Powell, Chaloupka and Bao 2007), and in communities of color, particularly in predominantly African American communities (Fleischhacker et al. 2011; Forsyth et al. 2012; Fraser et al. 2010; Kwate et al. 2009). Low-income, African American communities are an ideal location for fast food restaurants due to depressed land values, a less educated labor force, minimal retail competition, a captive customer base, and the lack of political capital to oppose their establishment (Fraser et al. 2010; Kwate 2008).

   While it is logical to assume that limiting fast food outlets would help to improve health outcomes for African Americans, this strategy could indirectly perpetuate negative health outcomes by removing a source of employment (Kwate 2008). Fast food or limited-service restaurants are a major employer in the U.S., employing over 3.5 million people in close to 225,000 outlets across the nation in 2012. On average, each fast food establishment employed 16 people and generated

$826,000 in sales (U.S. Census Bureau 2012). They can also provide an entry into the workforce for more than just teenagers given that the average age of a fast food employee is 28 (Surbey 2014). Conversely, while fast food restaurants can be lucrative for some at senior levels, most outlets have low profit margins and cut costs by hiring unskilled labor. Fast food jobs tend to be part-time and low paying, on average $8.69 an hour. It is estimated that 20 percent of front line workers live in households that earn less than the federal poverty line and 23 percent are within the limit to be eligible for public assistance programs. Additionally, only 13 percent receive health benefits through their employer (Allegretto 2013). A recent study estimated that 52 percent of front line fast food workers, excluding managerial positions, participate in at least one public assistance program (Allegretto 2013). In this regard, critics argue that fast food outlets contribute to the perpetuation of socioeconomically stratified communities by keeping wages depressed.

This minimal investment in employees is carried through to the investment fast food restaurants make in the local economy. The return on investment to the local community from franchise chain fast food restaurants is lower than that of other locally owned establishments. Recent studies estimate that local retail and restaurants return significantly more revenue to the local community than chain retail and restaurants. One study estimates that chain restaurants return only 37 percent of revenue to the local community whereas non-chain local restaurants return 56 percent (Mitchell 2014). Yet, while fast food outlets are a less-than-ideal option for community wellbeing, they do play a role in the economic and social aspects of the wellbeing of depressed communities with minimal opportunities, resources and political capital to advocate for alternative options. Fast food outlets can serve as potential drivers of economic development for a community by choosing to invest in the community and in hiring from the local labor force (Kwate 2008). Addressing public health concerns in communities of color and low-income areas require addressing the underlying issues of poverty, not their symptoms.

Zoning for public health: right tool for the right job

An alternative solution for investment to address public health concerns in communities of color and of low-income is to expand, rather than restrict, land uses to encourage supermarkets, particularly full-service, chain grocery stores. Research shows a strong association between supermarkets and weight, with improved access to supermarkets leading to intake of healthier food options (Cummins et al. 2005; Ford and Dzewaltowski 2008; Larson, Story and Nelson 2009) and reduced weight (Jeffery et al. 2006; Lopez, 2007; Viola et al. 2013). In a review of the literature on healthy food access, Larson, Story, and Nelson (2009) found that almost all of the studies reported that the greater the availability of supermarkets, the higher the intake of healthy foods and the lower the risk for obesity. One study found that the presence of a supermarket in a census tract is associated with a 9 percent lower prevalence of being overweight and a 24 percent lower prevalence of obesity (Morland, Wing, and Roux 2002). The addition of a supermarket can further decrease rates of overweight by 0.086 percent and obesity by 0.106 percent within a quarter-mile area, with an even greater impact for African American communities (Viola et al. 2013).

However, the availability of supermarkets is not equally distributed across communities. In a scan of zoning ordinances for 175 communities, low-income communities are less likely to permit uses that allow for supermarkets or other fresh produce outlets, like farmers' markets, than higher income communities (Chriqui et al. 2012). In a review of literature, Ford and Dzewaltowski (2008) discuss how geographic differences result in disparities in the retail food environment, particularly in neighborhoods of low socioeconomic status and communities of color and how exposure to areas lacking supermarkets can lead to higher rates of obesity. Supermarkets help to offset the association between weight and low socioeconomic status by increasing intake of healthy food options, especially in areas with high concentrations of communities of color (Larson, Story, and Nelson 2009). In census tracts with a higher proportion of African Americans, consumption of fruits and vegetables increased by 32 percent with each additional supermarket in the tract (Morland, Wing, and Roux 2002). These same associations with supermarkets cannot be conferred on other food retail establishments, like convenience stores or independent grocery stores, because they do not offer the same products, of the same quality, at the same price.

Given variations in association between health outcomes, food retail type, and neighborhood socioeconomic characteristics, local planning and zoning controls ought to be tailored to fit the context of a community. Based on their findings from a study on walkability and healthy food access in Salt Lake County, Utah, Zink et al. (2009) posit that, "neighborhood design interventions targeted at reducing obesity risk might be more effective if they are tailored to the residents' socioeconomic circumstances." Foundations, national policy organizations and cities are experimenting with locally derived neighborhood design interventions to address health disparities. The Robert Wood Johnson Foundation is working with the National League of Cities to pilot the Learning Collaborative on Health Disparities in seven cities to improve access to healthy food and opportunities for physical activity as a means to prevent childhood obesity. The Foundation is also working with the Health Impact Project to encourage state legislation that requires consideration of health effects in government policies, plans and projects. The Urban Land Institute's Building Healthy Places Initiative is piloting an effort to redesign select transportation corridors into healthy spaces in four cities. The infusion of interest and funding by national organizations to drive comprehensive local efforts may provide a bridge to affect the national problem of obesity through multifaceted local control solutions.

Price point: taxation

Zoning is not the only regulatory tool available to local jurisdictions to modify the food environment in the interest of public health. Altering the relative price of unhealthy food, like fast food or sugar-sweetened beverages, through a price increase or tax (sometimes called a junk or fat tax) is another strategy being explored by public health professionals to prevent obesity. Literature on the price elasticity of taxing unhealthy foods suggests that a tax or price increase on sodas has the most potential to impact health outcomes. Some analysts estimate that a 10 percent tax or increase in the price of soft drinks could reduce the purchase of sodas by 6.8 to 10 percent (Andreyeva 2010; Brownell and Freidan 2009) and the consumption of sodas by 3 percent (Duffey et al. 2010). Duffey et al. (2010) estimate that an 18 percent sales tax on sodas could decrease total energy intake for young adults by five pounds per person per year. In 2014, Mexico implemented a one peso per liter tax on sodas. A year later, this tax is showing an average decrease of 6 percent in soda purchases with an even higher decrease of 17 percent in purchases amongst those of the lowest-income (Sanger-Katz 2015). It is yet to be determined the impact that this tax will have on obesity rates. Increasing the price of sodas is also found to impact fast food consumption, particularly amongst African American males. Gordon-Larsen et al. (2011) estimate that a 20 percent increase in the price of soda could lead to African American males making 25 percent fewer visits to fast food outlets. However, extending price increases to other fast food items, like burgers, does not have a similar significant associated impact.

The drawback to taxing food is that it does not affect all populations equally. Amongst select populations, low-income populations and those already at risk for overweight or obesity, price increases tend to be more elastic (Powell and Chaloupka 2009). For low-income families, food taxes have a regressive impact since low-income families spend more of their household income on food. Ironically, a soda tax might have little effect on families that receive Supplemental Nutrition Assistance Benefits (SNAP), because food purchased with SNAP is not taxed (Chriqui et al. 2008; Powell and Chaloupka 2009). Whether to permit use of federal dollars to purchase unhealthy food, particularly soda, also is of debate amongst advocates and policy makers, with critics arguing that such taxes unfairly restrict the individual choice of SNAP recipients.

A powerful, and more equitable, combination that could change health outcomes for the general population, and at the same time help to improve the food landscape in low-income or communities of color, would be to use revenue from a soda or junk tax to subsidize double dollar or other incentive programs for fresh fruits and vegetables. In a review of literature on the price elasticity of fast food, Powell and Chaloupka (2009) conclude that there would need to be substantial changes in the price of fruits and vegetables to improve health outcomes significantly. Like with zoning, food taxes can also be detrimental to communities of color and low-income neighborhoods due to limited financial and community resources, unless paired with strategies that encourage healthier lifestyle choices.

Prioritizing outcomes

The relationship between the built environment and public health is complex – and we haven't even touched on physical activity. There is no one-size-fits-all strategy for addressing obesity, especially when it comes to modifying the built environment. While local governments have a number of regulatory tools that they can employ to address obesity, including zoning, taxes, and incentives, each tool and the community context must be carefully evaluated to fully understand the benefits and consequences to the community wellbeing.

As such, the question then becomes, what is the priority – individual health, public health, or community wellbeing? The priority might be all of the above, and the solution might be a comprehensive suite of tools that cross social, economic, health and political dimensions of a community's wellbeing. This type of change is slow and dispersed but can have lasting impact.

References

Abdollah, T. 2007. A strict order for fast food: The City Council may consider a moratorium on allowing new outlets in South L.A., where obesity rates are high. *Los Angeles Times*, September 10. Available online at http://articles.latimes.com/2007/sep/10/local/me-fastfood10 (accessed June 6, 2016).

Active Living Research. 2011. *Do All Children Have Places to Be Active? Disparities in Access to Physical Activity in Racial and Ethnic Minority and Lower-Income Communities.* Available online at http://activelivingresearch.org/files/Synthesis_Taylor-Lou_Disparities_Nov2011_0.pdf (accessed June 6, 2016).

Ahern, M., Brown, C., and Dukas, S. 2011. "A national study of the association between food environments and county-level health outcomes." *The Journal of Rural Health*, 27 (4): 367–379.

Allegretto, S.A., Doussard, M., Graham-Squire, D., Jacobs, K., Thompson, D., and Thompson, J. 2013. "Fast Food, Poverty Wages: The Public Cost of Low-Wage Jobs in the Fast Food Industry." *UC Berkeley Labor Center.* Available online at http://laborcenter.berkeley.edu/pdf/2013/fast_food_poverty_wages.pdf (accessed June 6, 2016).

Andreyeva, T., Long, M., and Brownell, K. 2010. "The impact of food prices on consumption: A systematic review of research on the price elasticity of demand for food." *American Journal of Public Health*, 100 (2): 216–222. Available online at DOI:10.2105/AJPH.2008.151415.

Acevedo-Garcia, D., and Lochner, K. 2003. *Residential Segregation and Health: Neighborhoods and Health.* New York: Oxford University Press, 265–287.

Binkley, J., Eales, J., and Jekanowski, M. 2000. "The relation between dietary change and rising U.S. obesity." *International Journal of Obesity*, 24: 1032–1039.

Block, J., Scribner, R., and De Salvo, K. 2004. "Fast food, race/ethnicity, and income: A geographic analysis." *American Journal of Preventive Medicine*, 27 (3): 211–7.

Boone-Heinonen, J., Gordon-Larsen, P., Kiefe, C.I., Shikany, J.M., Lewis, C.E., and Popkin, B.M. 2011. "Fast food restaurants and food stores: Longitudinal associations with diet in young adults: The CARDIA Study." *Archives of Internal Medicine*, 171 (13): 1162–1170.

Bowman, S., and Vinyard, B. 2004. "Fast food consumption of US adults: Impact on energy and nutrient intakes and overweight status." *Journal of the American College of Nutrition*, 23 (2): 163–8. Available online at DOI:10.1080/07315724.2004.10719357.

Brownell, K., and Frieden, T. 2009. "Ounces of prevention: The public policy case for taxes on sugared beverages." *New England Journal of Medicine*, 360: 1805–1808. Available online at DOI: 10.1056/NEJMp0902392, www.nejm.org/toc/nejm/360/18 (accessed June 6, 2016).

Centers for Disease Control and Prevention. 2011. *Impact of the Built Environment on Health.* Available online at www.cdc.gov/nceh/publications/factsheets/impactofthebuiltenvironmentonhealth.pdf (accessed September 7, 2016).

Chriqui, J.F., Eidson, S.S., Bates, H., Kowalczyk, S., and Chaloupka, F.J. 2008. "State sales tax rates for soft drinks and snacks sold through grocery stores and vending machines, 2007." *Journal of Public Health Policy*, 29: 226–249. Available online at DOI: 10.1057/jphp.2008.9 (accessed June 6, 2016).

Chriqui, J.F., Thrun, E., Rimkus, L., Barker, D.C., and Chaloupka, F.J. 2012. *Zoning for Healthy Food Access Varies by Community Income* – A BTG Research Brief. Bridging the Gap Program, Health Policy Center, Institute for Health Research and Policy, University of Illinois at Chicago. Available online at www.bridgingthegapresearch.org/_asset/n5qtpc/btg_food_zoning_final-0612.pdf. (accessed June 6, 2016).

Cobb, L.K., Appel, L.J., Franco, M., Jones-Smith, J.C., Nur, A., and Anderson, C.A. 2015. "The relationship of the local food environment with obesity: A systematic review of methods, study quality, and results." *Obesity*, 23 (7): 1331–1344.

Coburn, J. 2009. *Toward the Healthy City: People, Places and the Politics of Urban Planning.* Cambridge, MA: The MIT Press.

Cummins, S., Petticrew, M., Higgins, C., Findlay, A., and Sparks, L. 2005. "Large scale food retailing as an intervention for diet and health: Quasi-experimental evaluation of a natural experiment." *Journal of Epidemiology and Community Health*, 59 (12): 1035–1040.

Currie, J., DellaVigna, S., Moretti, E., and Pathania, V. 2010. "The effect of Fast food restaurants on obesity and weight gain." *American Economic Journal: Economic Policy*, 2 (3): 32–63. Available online at DOI: 10.1257/pol.2.3.32.

Cutler, D., Glaeser, E., and Shapiro, J. 2003. "Why have Americans become more obese?" *Journal of Economic Perspectives*, 17 (3): 93–118.

Duffey, K., and Popkin, B. 2011. "Energy density, portion size, and eating occasions: Contributions to increased energy intake in the United States, 1977–2006." *PLoS Medicine*, 8 (6): e1001050. Available online at DOI:10.1371/journal.pmed.1001050.

Duffey, K., Gordon-Larsen, P., Jacobs, D.R. Jr., Williams, O.D., and Popkin, B.M. 2007. "Differential associations of fast food and restaurant food consumption with 3-y change in body mass index: The Coronary Artery Risk Development in Young Adults Study." *American Journal of Clinical Nutrition*, 85 (1): 201–8.

Duffey, K., Gordon-Larsen, P., Shikany, J.M., Guilkey, D., Jacobs, D.R. Jr., and Popkin, B.M. 2010. "Food price and diet and health outcomes: 20 years of the CARDIA study." *Archives of Internal Medicine*, 170 (5): 420–426. Available online at DOI:10.1001/archinternmed.2009.545.

Dunn, R., Sharkey, J., and Horel, S. 2012. "The effect of fast-food availability on fast-food consumption and obesity among rural residents: An analysis by race/ethnicity." *Economics and Human Biology*, 10 (1): 1–13.

Fleischhacker, S.E., Evenson, K.R., Rodriguez, D.A., and Ammerman, A.S. 2011. "A systematic review of fast food access studies." *Obesity Reviews*, 12: e460–e471. Available online at DOI:10.1111/j.1467-789X.2010.00715.x.

Ford, P., and Dzewaltowski, D. 2008. "Disparities in obesity prevalence due to variation in the retail food environment: Three testable hypotheses." *Nutrition Review*, 66 (4): 216–28.

Forsyth, A., Wallb, M., Larsonc, N., Storyc, M., and Neumark-Sztainerc, D. 2012. "Do adolescents who live or go to school near fast food restaurants eat more frequently from fast food restaurants?" *Health and Place*, 18 (6): 1261–1269. Available online at DOI:10.1016/j.healthplace.2012.09.005.

Fraser, L., Edwards, K.L., Cade, J., and Clarke, G.P. 2010. "The geography of fast food outlets: A review." *International Journal of Environmental Research and Public Health*, 7 (5): 2290–2308. Available online at DOI:10.3390/ijerph7052290.

Freeman, A. 2007. "Fast food: Oppression through poor nutrition." *California Law Review*, 95: 2221–2259.

French, S.A., Story, M., Neumark-Sztainer, D., Fulkerson, J.A., and Hannan, P. 2001. "Fast food restaurant use among adolescents: Associations with nutrient intake, food choices and behavioral and psychosocial variables." *International Journal of Obesity*, 25 (12): 1823–1833. Available online at DOI: 10.1038/sj.ijo.0801820.

Globe Newswire. 2015. "Indoor Harvest Corp Set to Design-Build World's First Publicly-Owned, Open Data, Crowdfunded, Vertical Farm Research and Education Campus." Available online at http://globenewswire.com/news-release/2015/12/02/792403/0/en/Indoor-Harvest-Corp-Set-to-Design-Build-World-s-First-Publicly-Owned-Open-Data-Crowdfunded-Vertical-Farm-Research-and-Education-Campus.html (accessed June 6, 2016).

Gordon-Larsen, P. 2014. "Food availability/convenience and obesity." *Advanced Nutrition*, 5: 809–817. Available online at DOI: 10.3945/an.114.007070.

Gordon-Larsen, P., Guilkey, D., and Popkin, B. 2011. "An economic analysis of community-level fast food prices and individual-level fast food intake: Longitudinal effects." *Health and place*, 17 (6): 1235–1241. Available online at DOI:10.1016/j.healthplace.2011.07.011.

Hickson, D.A., Diez Roux, A.V., Smith, A.E., Tucker, K.L., Gore, L.D., Zhang, L., and Wyatt, S.B. 2011. "The associations of fast food restaurant availability with dietary intake and weight among African Americans in the Jackson Heart Study, 2000–2004." *American Journal of Public Health*, 101 (Suppl. 1): S301–S309. Available online at DOI:10.2105/AJPH.2010.300006.

Hu, F. 2008. *Obesity Epidemiology*. Boston, MA: Oxford University Press.

Jeffery, R., Baxter, J., McGuire, M., and Linde, J. 2006. "Are fast food restaurants an environmental risk factor for obesity?" *The International Journal of Behavioral Nutrition and Physical Activity*, 3, 2. Available online at DOI:10.1186/1479–5868–3-2.

Kwate, N. 2008. "Fried chicken and fresh apples: Racial segregation as a fundamental cause of fast food density in black neighborhoods." *Health and Place*, 14 (1): 32–44. Available online at DOI: 10.1016/j.healthplace.2007.04.001.

Kwate, N., Yau, C.Y., Loh, J.M., and Williams, D. 2009. "Inequality in obesigenic environments: Fast food density in New York City." *Health and Place*, 15 (1): 364–373.

Landrine, H., and Corral, I. 2009. "Separate and unequal: Residential segregation and black health disparities." *Ethnicity and Disease*, 19 (2): 179.

Larson, N., Story, M., and Nelson, M. 2009. "Neighborhood environments: Disparities in access to healthy foods in the U.S." *American Journal of Preventive Medicine*, 36 (1): 74–81. Available online at DOI: 10.1016/j.amepre.2008.09.025.

Lopez, R. 2007. "Neighborhood risk factors for obesity." *Obesity*, 15: 2111–2119.

Maddock, J. 2004. "The relationship between obesity and the prevalence of fast-food restaurants: State-level analysis." *American Journal of Health Promotion*, 19: 137–43.

Mitchell, S. 2014. "Key studies: Why local matters." *Institute for Local Self-Reliance*. Available online at http://ilsr.org/key-studies-walmart-and-bigbox-retail/ (accessed June 6, 2016).

Morland, K., Wing, S., and Roux, A. 2002. "The contextual effect of the local food environment on residents' diets: The atherosclerosis risk in communities study." *American Journal of Public Health*, 92 (11): 1761–1768.

Neckerman, K., Bader, M., Purciel, M., and Yousefzadeh, P. 2009. "Measuring food access in urban areas." Available online at www.npc.umich.edu/news/events/food-access/ neckerman_et_al.pdf (accessed June 6, 2016).

Nolan, J., and Salkin, P. 2007. *Land Use in a Nutshell.* St. Paul, MN: West Academic Publishing.

Ogden, C.L., Carroll, M.D., Kit, B.K., and Flegal, K.M. 2014. "Prevalence of childhood and adult obesity in the United States, 2011–2012." *Journal of the American Medical Association,* 311 (8): 806–814. Available online at DOI:10.1001/jama.2014.732.

Pereira, M.A., Kartashov, A.I., Ebbeling, C.B., Van Horn, L., Slattery, M.L., Jacobs, D.R. Jr., and Ludwig, D.S. 2005. "Fast-food habits, weight gain, and insulin resistance (the CARDIA study): 15-year prospective analysis." *The Lancet,* 365 (9453): 36–42.

Pollard, J., Kirk, S., and Cade, J. 2002. "Factors affecting food choice in relation to fruit and vegetable intake: A review." *Nutrition Research Reviews,* 15: 373–387 Available online at DOI:10.1079/NRR200244.

Powell, L., and Chaloupka, F. 2009. "Food prices and obesity: Evidence and policy implications for taxes and subsidies." *The Milbank Quarterly,* 87 (1): 229–257.

Powell, L., Chaloupka, F., and Bao, Y. 2007. "The availability of fast-food and full-service restaurants in the United States: Associations with neighborhood characteristics." *American Journal of Preventive Medicine,* 33 (4 Suppl): S240–S245.

Prentice, A., and Jebb, S. 2003. "Fast foods, energy density and obesity: A possible mechanistic link." *Obesity Reviews,* 4: 187–194. Available online at DOI: 10.1046/j.1467–789X.2003.00117.x.

Remington, P., Brownson, R., and Wegner, M. 2010. *Chronic Disease Epidemiology and Control.* Washington, DC: American Public Health Association.

Richardson, A., Boone-Heinonen, J., Popkin, B.M., and Gordon-Larsen, P. 2011. "Neighborhood fast food restaurants and fast food consumption: A national study." *BMC Public Health,* 11 (543).

Rossen, L., and Pollack, K. 2012. "Making the connection between zoning and health disparities." *Environmental Justice,* 5 (3): 119–127.

Rosenheck, R. (2008). Fast food consumption and increased caloric intake: A systematic review of a trajectory towards weight gain and obesity risk. *Obesity Reviews,* 9: 535–547. Available online at DOI:10.1111/j.1467–789X.2008.00477.x.

Rothman, K., Greenland, S., and Lash, T. 2008. *Modern Epidemiology,* 3rd Edition. Philadelphia, PA: Lippincott, Williams and Wilkins.

Sanger-Katz, M. 2015. "Yes, Soda Taxes Do Seem to Discourage Soda Drinking." *New York Times,* October 13, 2015. Available online at http://www.nytimes.com/2015/10/13/ upshot/yes-soda-taxes-seem-to-cut-soda-drinking.html?_r=0 (accessed June 6, 2016).

Silver, C. 1997. "The racial origins of zoning in American cities." In June Manning Thomas and Marsha Ritzdorf (eds.), *Urban Planning and the African American Community: In the shadows.* Thousand Oaks, CA: Sage Publications, 23–42.

Surbey, J. 2014. Fast Food Myth and Wages. *U.S. Department of Labor Blog.* Available online at http://blog.dol.gov/2014/12/11/fast-food-myths-and-wages/ (accessed June 6, 2016).

Sturm, R., and Cohen, D. 2009. "Zoning for health? The year old ban on new fast food restaurants in south L.A." *Health Affects* 28 (6): 1088–1097.

Sturm, R., and Hattori, A. 2015. "Diet and obesity in Los Angeles County 2007–2012: Is there a measurable effect of the 2008 'Fast-Food Ban'?" *Social Science and Medicine.* Available online at http://dx.DOI.org/10.1016/j.socscimed.2015.03.004 (accessed September 7, 2016).

U.S. Census Bureau Economic Census and Population Estimates. 2012. *Industry Snapshots – Limited-Service Restaurants (NAICS 722513)*. Available online at http://thedataweb. rm.census.gov/TheDataWeb_HotReport2/econsnapshot/2012/snapshot. hrml?NAICS=722513 (accessed June 6, 2016).

Viola, D., Arno, P.S., Maroko, A.R., Schechter, C.B., Sohler, N., Rundle, A., Neckerman, K.M., and Maantay, J. 2013. "Overweight and obesity: Can we reconcile evidence about supermarkets and fast food retailers for public health policy?" *Journal of Public Health Policy*, 34: 424–438.

Wiseman, J., and Brasher, K. 2008. "Community wellbeing in an unwell world: Trends, challenges, and possibilities." *Journal of Public Health Policy*, 29: 353–366.

5 From food access to food justice

A case study of the Somerville Mobile Farmers' Market

*Sara Shostak, Janaki Blum, Chris Mancini,
Luisa Oliveira, Lisa Robinson, and
Erica Satin-Hernandez*

In October 2015, U.S. Secretary of Agriculture Tom Vilsack announced $8.1 million in grants for projects in 23 states to enhance the effectiveness of Supplemental Nutrition Assistance Program (SNAP) operations at farmers' markets, including "staff training and technical assistance, creating educational materials, and raising awareness among current SNAP participants that their benefits may be used to purchase the healthy, fresh foods at these outlets."[1] According to the press release about the new funding, "Today's announcement is part of a USDA-wide effort to support President Obama's commitment to strengthening local and regional food systems ... [and] to boost affordable access to local, fresh and healthy foods, which ... benefits the health of all Americans, regardless of income levels." One of the Healthy People 2020 goals is to increase fruit and vegetable consumption among *all* U.S. populations. Meeting this public health goal will require interventions that improve access to fruits and vegetables, especially for individuals living in low-income communities and communities of color (Morland 2007; Moore and Diez-Roux 2006).

A robust literature demonstrates that people living in low-income communities and communities of color are less likely to have access to a fully stocked grocery store (Morland, et al. 2002, 2006; Morland and Evenson 2009; Walker, Keane and Burke 2010; Zenk, et al. 2005); additionally, the availability of chain supermarkets in Black neighborhoods is less than that in their White counterparts, even when controlling for neighborhood income (Powell, et al. 2007). Grocery stores located in low-income communities tend to carry produce of less variety and lower quality, when compared to stores in more affluent communities (Latham and Moffat 2007). At the same time, low-income urban communities are more likely to have abundant fast food outlets and convenience stores (Block, et al. 2004; Freudenberg and Galea 2008), where food is typically both more expensive and less healthy (Latham and Moffatt 2007). Consequently, scholars and policy makers characterize these neighborhoods as *food deserts* – "area[s] with limited access to affordable and nutritious foods, particularly such an area composed of predominantly lower income neighborhoods and communities" (USDA 2009).[2]

However, recent scholarship on the food environment and diet has found that improving the simple *availability* of healthy food in a specific geographic area is not enough to change individuals' purchasing and dietary behaviors (Cummins, et al. 2014; Elbel, et al, 2015; LeDoux and Vojnovic 2013). This research indicates that the lived experience of a food environment is shaped also not only by availability, but by *accessibility* – "the location of the food supply and ease of getting to that location;" *affordability* – "food prices and people's perceptions of worth relative to the cost;" *acceptability* – "people's attitudes about … whether the given supply of products meets their personal standards;" and *accommodation* – "how well local food sources accept and adapt to local residents' needs" (Caspi, et al. 2012b: 1173). As such, researchers have suggested that food access may not be well captured by objective measures of geographic distance to markets. Rather, it is shaped by more subjective factors, such as the *perceived* distance to markets (Caspi, et al. 2012a) and relationships between customers and store owners (Cannuscio, et al. 2010). Related, the *foodways* of residents, which refers to sociocultural processes and preferences regarding "how and what communities eat, where and how they shop and what motivates their food preferences" may mediate the effects of the food environment (Alkon, et al. 2013: 127; see also Cannuscio, et al. 2010). Fully understanding issues of food access requires consideration of social and cultural dynamics, as well as aspects of the built environment. Importantly, this refocuses our attention on the agency, preferences, cultures, and relationships of people buying food for themselves and their families.

This expanded focus aligns public health concerns more closely with issues of food justice. Food justice advocates, at both the community and the national level, have argued that communities have "the right to grow, sell, and eat [food that is] nutritious, affordable, culturally appropriate, and grown locally with care for the well-being of the land, workers, and animals" (Alkon and Agyeman 2011: 5). How we produce and achieve equitable access to healthy food can thus be understood as a matter of both public health and social justice.

The jumping off point for this chapter is the broad question of whether, and how, farmers' markets may address these important concerns. As we describe below, the literature on the public health and social justice contributions of farmers' markets is mixed, especially from the perspective of food justice; additionally, despite their growing popularity, mobile markets remain virtually unstudied. Our analysis comes from a case study of the Somerville Mobile Farmers' Market (SMFM), a summer season market that brings fresh produce into low-income communities in Somerville, Massachusetts. Based on interviews, ethnographic observation, attendance counts, and sales and survey data, we identify the contributions the Market has made and the challenges it faces. Our conclusions point to next steps for meeting the interrelated goals of improving public health and advancing food justice in low-income communities.

Farmers' markets, public health, and social justice

In 2011, the Centers for Disease Control and Prevention included "Start or expand farmers' markets in all settings" among its strategies for increasing fruit and vegetable consumption in the U.S. population (CDC 2011: 21). In its advocacy for this approach, the CDC noted the relative ease of setting up a seasonal farmers' market (as compared to a supermarket) and highlighted the particular benefits of farmers' markets in food deserts, commenting that "residents of low-income neighborhoods, where supermarkets are scarce and the small grocery and convenience stores that do exist sell limited fresh produce, may benefit most from the access to fruits and vegetables provided through farmers' markets" (CDC 2011: 21).

At this time, there is only a limited literature on whether farmers' markets increase fruit and vegetable consumption in low-income communities and communities of color (McCormack, et al. 2010). Research has more often focused on the effects of providing low-income consumers with economic incentives for shopping at farmers' markets (Baronberg, et al. 2013; Freedman, et al. 2014; Young, et al. 2013). This is important because concern about the cost of food has been identified as a barrier to shopping at farmers' markets (Zepeda 2009; Kato and McKinney 2014; Ruelas, et al. 2012). However, a study that assessed the effects of introducing farmers' markets into low-income and racially diverse communities found that the markets increased both fruit and vegetable consumption and the *perceived importance* of fruit and vegetable consumption among residents (Evans, et al. 2012). In a study of a farmers' market in a low-income community in Chicago, residents reported higher rates of satisfaction with the fresh fruits and vegetables provided by the market as compared to the access, quality, variety, and prices of products available to them year round through local stores (Suarez-Balcazar, et al. 2006).

A few studies find other positive effects. For example, research suggests that farmers' markets can contribute to low-income communities by serving as venues for health promotion and other educational and social activities, which in turn may foster community and build relationships among residents (Zepeda, et al. 2014; Holben 2011). Further, in urban food deserts, where there are limited venues for purchasing fresh fruits and vegetables, the introduction of farmers' markets may create enough competition to drive down the cost of produce for consumers shopping at local stores (Larsen and Gilliland 2009).

The literature on mobile markets, in particular, is quite sparse, and evinces mixed evidence for their effects. Research suggests that the capacity of mobile markets to travel, and therefore serve a wider geographic area, may give them an advantage, relative to brick-and-mortar stores, in increasing fruit and vegetable consumption in low-income communities (Widener, et al. 2012). Some studies have found increases in fruit consumption among children (Tester, et al. 2012) and vegetable consumption among seniors (Abusabha, et al. 2011) associated with mobile markets. However, evaluation of mobile markets in Philadelphia found very limited utilization in target communities (Philadelphia

Greensgrow Project 2012). Intriguingly, one study found that health status (i.e., how people perceive their health) is associated with access to a mobile market, even when there were no observable improvements in traditional biomedical measures of health status (i.e., BMI, blood pressure and blood sugar) (Lewis and Zollinger 2012). Zepeda and colleagues (2014) suggest that building trusting relationships and communicating to shoppers that mobile markets are nonprofits committed to improving food access can improve their reception and utilization in low-income communities.

Farmers' markets have also been a focus of critiques, especially on issues of food justice. To begin, critics point out that the typical farmers' market customer is white, middle to upper class, and well educated (Brown 2002; Zepeda 2009); likewise, most farmers markets are located in relatively privileged communities and often serve consumers who have the time, money, and identity politics that support engagement with resource intensive alternative food practices (Guthman 2008). Accordingly, scholars have argued that the "whiteness" of farmers' market exclude people of color, thereby limiting their potential to advance public health or social justice goals (Alkon and McCullen 2010; Slocum 2007). A second critique centers on the possibility that efforts to bring fresh fruits and vegetables to low-income communities represents a new form of paternalism. Of particular concern is the possibility that focusing on food consumption individualizes responsibility for personal and population health, and elides a number of structural factors, including poverty and access to health care, which may be more consequential for population health (Lyson 2014). A third, and related, critique contends that positioning farmers' markets as a strategy to address issues of food access and public health recapitulates the neoliberal "prescription" that social problems must be resolved through market relations (Alkon and McCullen 2010: 939) and individual consumer behavior (Lyson 2014). The concern here is that voluntary organizations and markets are being asked to fulfill the obligations of the state to its citizens, e.g., to provide food for those who cannot afford it without assistance (Alkon and Mares 2012: 348). Scholars writing from this political economic perspective call for collective social action to transform conventional agriculture (Guthman 2008) and/or remediate the economic policies that lead to poverty, food insecurity, and health inequalities (Alkon and Mares 2012). However, some critics allow for a role for farmers' markets in such transformation, noting that "farmers markets have the potential to act as entry points for more progressive, politicized social movement activity" (Alkon and McCullen 2010: 941).

The role and capacity of farmers' markets in general, and mobile markets in particular, to advance public health and social justice goals are timely concerns, especially as markets have surged in popularity. In the past ten years, the number of farmers' markets in the United States has more than doubled, from 3,706 in 2004 to 8,268 in 2014.[3] The Commonwealth of Massachusetts is home to nearly 300 farmers' markets, a dramatic increase from the 8 operating in 1979.[4] According to the United States Department of Agriculture (USDA), Massachusetts ranks seventh in the nation in the number of farmer's markets.[5] Somerville is one of several municipalities in Massachusetts that hosts a mobile market, that is, a market that travels to communities where there is less access to healthy food, bringing fruits and vegetables "to the doorsteps" of low-income individuals and families.

Research questions, data, and methods

In 2014, following a review and approval from the Brandeis University Committee for the Protection of Human Subjects in Research, we conducted an evaluation of the Somerville Mobile Farmers' Market oriented to the following sets of questions: 1) Who is shopping at the SMFM? Where do they live? Where else do they shop?; 2) From the perspectives of customers, in what ways is the SMFM succeeding and in what ways could the SMFM be improved?; 3) What lessons can be learned from the SMFM in regard to efforts to increase food access and food justice?

More broadly, the case study reported here draws on a mixed-methods approach. The data gathered include the following:

1 *Interviews with the market organizers* were conducted by two authors (SS and JB), recorded and transcribed verbatim.
2 *Attendance counts and sales data* were generated by two authors (JB and ESH). These include SNAP/EBT sales, which provide a means of assessing whether, or to what extent, low-income customers are shopping at the SMFM.
3 *Dot Surveys and open-ended questions*, conducted by two authors (SS and JB) and youth from the Groundwork Somerville Green Team[6] at the SMFM for the entirety (4 hours) of four separate Markets, from June to September 2014.[7] These data came from using the techniques of Rapid Market Assessment (Lev, et al. 2008), developed to conduct research in the (ideally) busy public setting of a farmers' market. Because these are relatively novel research methods, we describe them in some detail.

Dot surveys were set up on a fence across from the market. Each question was written in large print on a piece of butcher paper. As customers exited the market, we invited them to participate if they had not done so previously. Individuals who agreed to participate were given a sheet of colored stickers (dots) and asked to place their dots next to the best answers to the following questions. Although the survey questions were written in English, we provided translation to the best of our ability, drawing on our own language skills and those of other volunteers at the Market.

The dot survey posed closed-answer questions, which were arrayed in a different order each time the survey was conducted: *1) Where do you live?; 2) How often do you come to the market?; 3) Does the market help you – or your children – eat more fruits and vegetables?; 4) How did you hear about the market?; 5) Why do you shop at the market?; 6) Where else do you shop for food?* Answers to the dot survey data were tabulated by an author with the assistance of the Groundwork Somerville Green Team, and appear below as descriptive quantitative data.

Additionally, each day we did a dot survey we also asked market customers to answer three following open-ended questions: *1) What do you like about the market?; 2) How could the market be improved?; 3) What other items would you like to be able to purchase at the Market?* The answers to these questions were recorded on large sheets of butcher paper by the authors (SS and JB) or one of the youth from the Green Team, who also assisted with translation. These answers were entered into Excel, which allowed us to group them by theme and tabulate frequencies.

4   *Ethnographic observation*, conducted by one author (SS). The periods of observation included the four days on which we were conducting surveys and two days when the author attended the market as a customer. Following each period of observation, the author wrote up field notes to capture her direct observations (Emerson, Fretz, and Shaw 1995) and memos to record her reflections on what she had observed (Charmaz 2006).

Such a combination of methods is not uncommon in studies of farmers' markets (e.g., Freedman, et al. 2014; Kato and McKinney 2014). Indeed, we contend that a mixed-methods approach is the only way to begin to address the array of objective and subjective factors that are theorized to constitute food access. Quantitative data were analyzed using basic descriptive statistics, while qualitative data were analyzed using the principles of grounded theory (Charmaz 2006).

Locating the Somerville Mobile Farmers' Market

Somerville is a mid-sized city located in Middlesex County, Massachusetts, approximately 2 miles north of Boston. With a population of 75,674 and a size of slightly more than 4 square miles, Somerville is the most densely populated community in New England. It is also strikingly diverse ethnically. Earlier waves of immigration brought families from Italy and Ireland. More recently, immigrants have arrived from Brazil, Haiti, Central America, and South East Asia (Ostrander 2013). According to census data, 25 percent of the city's residents (2009-2013) were born outside the United States and 32 percent of households report speaking a language other than English at home. More than 50 languages are spoken in the Somerville public schools.[8]

There is significant income inequality across the city. Although the median household income is $67,118, just over 15 percent of the city's residents live below the poverty line. East Somerville is home to many of the City's low-income residents. However, the Clarendon Hills Housing Project, in West Somerville, contains the most concentrated poverty in the City. Recent immigrants also are disproportionately concentrated in East Somerville.

Much of our data come from the residents of Mystic Housing Development, in East Somerville, which includes the Mystic River Development, a 240 unit state family housing development, and the Mystic View, a 215-unit federal family housing development. In 2012, 62 percent of families at the Mystic Housing Development earned less than $20,000 per year, which is less than half of the median household income of the census tract in which it is located, and less than one-third of the city's median household income. Seventy-eight percent of residents of the Mystic are non-white. Although there are numerous convenience stores within close walking distance, the closest grocery store can be accessed only by what residents describe as an "infrequent" and "unreliable" bus or by walking alongside a major highway. Residents report that they more often shop at Market Basket, a regional chain known for its low costs, which requires (round trip) either a 3-mile walk or 60+ minute commute via public transportation; while cabs are available, they are an expensive transportation option.

The SMFM has been held at the Mystic since it was founded in 2011. Its mission is to bring fresh fruit and vegetables to low-income residents of the city. The idea of a mobile market emerged out of conversations between Shape Up Somerville and organizations serving immigrant youth and families in the City:

> this was around the time that [the] Star Market had closed on Broadway, so there was this gap in access to food in that neighborhood. So we were talking … about how to [help] people to get to markets and to get to farmers' markets, and there were all these barriers that were coming up, like transportation, affordability … And then one of the youth from LIPS[9] said, "Why don't we just bring the produce directly to the people here in the housing development?" And so that's how it got started.
>
> (Interview 08).

In 2014, the SMFM operated from June through the end of October, at three locations over two days. On Thursdays, the Market was held first at the Somerville Council on Aging, near Davis Square; it then moved to the North Street Housing Project, in West Somerville. On Saturdays, it was at the Mystic Housing Development, in East Somerville. In 2014, there were two vendors at the SMFM. The primary vendor is Enterprise Farms, an organic farm located 100 miles away in Western Massachusetts. Additionally, the youth from the Groundwork Somerville Green Team, a green job skills development program, sell vegetables (and sometimes seedlings) that they grow at South Street, Somerville's first urban farm.

The SMFM is organized by Shape Up Somerville and Groundwork Somerville. Shape Up is a part of the City's Department of Health and Human Services where it pursues "a focus on the health and well-being of Somerville's most vulnerable residents, particularly a focus on health disparities and immigrant populations" (SUS 2013: 20). Groundwork Somerville is a community based organization that supports environmental stewardship, youth development, and urban agriculture. The SMFM has been supported by grants from the U.S. Centers for Disease Control and Prevention, the Massachusetts Department of Agriculture (MDAR), Mass in Motion, and private foundations, such as Project Bread and the Walmart Foundation. All proceeds from the Market go directly to the vendors; the market manager's salary is supported through grant funding, and volunteers and interns help with setting up, taking down, and evaluating the market.

Findings

We report findings organized along the three major themes that emerged from analysis of our data: 1) food availability and access; 2) the emerging importance of the SMFM as a community spacep; and 3) ongoing challenges to the SMFM to meet the demands of a diverse, multi-ethnic clientele, many who value familiar and culturally appropriate foods over "local" produce. We then discuss the restructuring of the Market, based on these findings, for the summer 2015 season.

Food availability and access

The SMFM is first and foremost a food access project. It has taken SNAP/EBT since its inception in 2011, and also accepts coupons from the WIC Farmers' Market Nutrition Program and the Seniors' Farmers' Market Nutrition Program. Produce is sold at what the organizers estimate to be wholesale rates, and residents from the housing developments are eligible to pay half the reduced rate on their purchases. This is the SMFM's equivalent of the dollar-to-dollar "match," which is common at other local farmers' markets, typically up to $5 or $10 of purchases. However, in contrast to other markets, there is no certification process for the 50 percent discount/ match at the SMFM: "We don't ask for ID because that is a scary prospect for some shoppers who may be undocumented" (Interview 09). Rather, customers are "on their honor" to report to the Market manager whether they are eligible.

In 2014, we counted an average of 52 unique groups/day purchasing produce at Saturday Market at the Mystic. According to the dot survey data, approximately 60 percent of shoppers at the Mystic Market live in the housing development, and nearly half shop there every week. Based on our conversations about language preferences with customers completing surveys at the Market, we know that it serves individuals who migrated from Haiti, the Dominican Republic, Bangladesh, Vietnam, and countries in Central America; while White and African American customers shop at the Market, recent immigrants appear to be the largest proportion of the clientele.

In 2014, the SMFM made direct sales of $10,916 of produce. This included sales paid for with coupons ($1,309), EBT/SNAP ($1,994), cash ($6,307) and debit and credit card payments ($1,306). The sales eligible for matching funds totaled $7,127. Consequently, the full value of the produce sold at the SMFM in 2014 was $18,044. Although the other two farmers' markets in Somerville also accept SNAP/EBT, the SMFM makes more SNAP/EBT sales than those markets combined (which reported $7,000 and $4,300 of SNAP/EBT sales, respectively, in 2014). Put differently, in 2014, just over 60 percent of the SNAP/EBT sales at the three Somerville Farmers' Markets were made at the relatively small SMFM; it is clearly meeting a need among the City's low-income residents.

Participants in the dot surveys report that the prices (33 percent), quality of the produce (30 percent), and location of the market (25 percent) are their top three reasons for shopping at the market. When asked open-ended questions about what they like about the SMFM, shoppers' responses were less constrained and, unsurprisingly, more varied. However, the quality (often "freshness") of the produce, reasonable prices, and convenient location were still the most frequently mentioned positive attributes of the market (n=140). Eighty-one percent of customers surveyed at the Mystic Market, on Saturdays, reported that the market helps them – or their children – eat more fruits and vegetables.

Community space

Alongside improving food access, the SMFM aims to provide a "community space" for its customers. A variety of community groups, including health and environmental organizations, gardening groups, and bike repair providers, have set up tables throughout the season. There are often boxes of free books, for both children and adults, and free merchandise from the SMFM sponsors that support activity at the market (e.g., mini-soccer balls, which were a huge hit with the kids). Additionally, Somerville's Food Day celebration was held at the Mystic, and included the Somerville Arts Council's bus (with a variety of activities for children), a second line brass band, a worm composting bin building table, and Brazilian music. Children at the Mystic seemed particularly thrilled with the arts and musical activities. During the brass band performance, a young girl rushed up to one author (SS) and declared, "I never knew before where songs come from!"

The market manager plays an important role at the SMFM. She is a resident of the Mystic Housing Development (the site of the Saturday market), who personally knows many of the customers. In addition to managing the busy queues of shoppers, making sales, and tracking purchases, she fields a staggering array of questions, not only about how to prepare specific vegetables, but also about ESL classes, local programs for youth, and other community resources. The Groundwork Somerville table is staffed by the local youth who have grown the produce they are selling. The structure of the SMFM means that customers are interacting with their peers and neighbors.

The commitment to creating a "community space" and providing mechanisms for community feedback has contributed to the development of the SMFM over time. The organizers are frank about how important it has been to reformulate the Market, in response to community preferences. They cite, for example an early "failure" of efforts to distribute vegetables using a subsidized community supported agriculture (CSA) model: "We thought it was a great idea … you just get a box every week. And it was so cheap … much cheaper than when you buy at the market" (Interview 08). However, the residents at the housing developments did not like this model at all: "They were like 'No, we want to pick out our produce. We want to see it. We don't want it in a box. We want to shop for it.' So we had to scrap it [the CSA]" (Interview 08). It was replaced with a regular farmers' market. The second reformulation, which is being undertaken in response to the 2014 evaluation data, highlights the difference between access and availability, on the one hand, and acceptability and accommodation, on the other (Caspi, et al. 2012b: 1173).

Market values

When asked what could be done to improve the market, respondents told us clearly that they wanted to be able to buy a wider variety of products. Alongside frequent requests for fruit, described in more detail below, we recorded requests for beans, meats, fish, honey, maple syrup, bread and other baked goods, and more and different vegetables. As one of the market organizers acknowledged "that's a challenge for us ... because a lot of times, we don't have the foods that they [shoppers] want" (Interview 08).

The sourcing model for the 2014 SMFM posed two particular challenges. First, as suggested by the feedback above, the only products available at the SMFM were fruits and vegetables. Second, the main vendor, Enterprise Farms, grows vegetables primarily for its large CSA program, which is not oriented to individuals from the diverse ethnic communities that shop at the SMFM. Consequently, many of the vegetables available were unfamiliar to the shoppers at the market. We repeatedly heard questions about how to cook lettuce from people from countries where greens are more often cooked; likewise, the appearance of garlic scapes provoked much amused discussion ("What do you *do* with these?"). In contrast, during the few weeks that callaloo – a green that is the central ingredient of the Caribbean dish of the same name, and also popular among South Asian cooks – was for sale, customers bought as much as they could carry, pulled out their phones to call their friends to tell them it was available, and expressed profound disappointment when it sold out. One week, the entire supply of callaloo sold out within the first ten minutes of the opening of the Market. The following week, women were queued nearly an hour before the opening of the Market, in hopes that callaloo would again be available.

Further, the emphasis of farmers' markets on selling *local* produce, defined by most Massachusetts farmers' markets as food grown by farmers in Massachusetts, constrains their ability to meet needs of shoppers who wish to eat decidedly non-local products. This tension was made most vivid in regard to customers' requests for fruit. When we asked SMFM customers "what else would you like to buy at the market?" nearly half of their requests (68 of 141 responses) were for more fruit. This desire was borne out by consumer behavior; when fruit (e.g., pints of strawberries) became available, it invariably sold out quickly. However, many shoppers specifically expressed a desire to purchase tropical fruits – bananas, guava, mangoes, pineapples – that are not grown locally. Likewise, they requested spices and herbs, such as turmeric and lemongrass, important to the cuisines of their countries of origin. Respondents knew that they were asking for non-local foods. One survey respondent stated explicitly, "I want things that are not grown here." Another shopper commented that she liked it when she saw vegetables similar to what she used to buy in Bangladesh. Yet another shopper asked if the Market could "import from other parts of the country."

The challenges at the SMFM point to the importance of aligning strategies for improving food access and affordability with more subjective aspects of the food environment, such as acceptability and accommodation. Ongoing feedback mechanisms at Markets are critical insofar as they allow customers to articulate such needs and preferences.

Lessons learned – and the 2015 season

As part of its ongoing commitment to be responsive to community needs, the SMFM changed its sourcing model for the 2015 summer season. Meeting the demand for fruit and more culturally relevant vegetables required that the SMFM organizers establish partnerships with new farms. The 2015 SMFM kept its partnerships with Enterprise Farm and Groundwork Somerville's urban farm, but added Kimball Fruit Farm, which specializes in various fruits, and World Farmers/ Flats Mentor Farm, a nonprofit where diverse immigrant farmers produce vegetables familiar to their home countries. Each of these partnerships filled a unique need for the SMFM, providing staple vegetables, culturally relevant produce, hyper-local specialty items, and fruit.

This new sourcing model, in turn, required that the City set up an account for the SMFM with its own EBT/debit/credit machine. The Market organizers report that this was a time intensive process. However, they consider the new market structure to be a success and a step towards financial sustainability, especially as the new aggregation system allows them increased control over the type and quantity of produce, as well as pricing. This has resulted in less underwriting of the produce and a better profit/loss rate.

With these new partnerships and EBT/SNAP account, the SMFM also was able to implement a new pricing structure, designed to support the market and its vendors while sustaining affordable prices for low-income consumers. Customers using the EBT match program, residents of the housing developments, and individuals shopping with WIC or seniors coupons continued to pay half of a wholesale rate. However, customers not using EBT/SNAP now pay what the market organizers describe as "a reasonable retail rate," which approximates the prices at Market Basket, a popular source of affordable produce in the City. Customers paying retail thereby support the EBT match program to increase the sustainability and self-sufficiency of the SMFM. This model is similar to the "subsidized CSA" programs being implemented by farms and food hubs in Massachusetts.[10] It also supported the extension of the Market to new sites, including a community library in a neighborhood with many low-income and immigrant families, a public school with high free and reduced lunch rates, a local bar and brewery, and a subsidized housing development for seniors and low-income families.

As the 2015 season was still underway at the time of this writing, we are not able to report on total sales for the season. However, it is already clear that, as anticipated, selling fruit at the SMFM has been a great success. In 2015, the market sold raspberries, blueberries, blackberries, grapes, peaches, and apples. Customers reported being happy with the fruit, which sold out every week, generating significant sales for the market.

Conclusions

Recent studies have reported that merely bringing healthy food into "food deserts," i.e., by building a supermarket, does not change the shopping or dietary behaviors of local residents (Elbel, et al. 2015). While these findings are surprising to those who focus primarily on issues of food availability and access, they are far less surprising from the perspective of food justice, which emphasizes honoring cultural traditions and giving shoppers a voice in deciding what and how products will be made available. Similarly, our data suggest that it is critical to the success of food access projects, such as mobile markets, to ask low-income consumers about their food preferences. The SMFM's reorganization, in response to the 2014 evaluation, points to the possibility that mobile markets can be flexible and responsive to the needs of low-income and immigrant shoppers.

This study also points to the possibility that farmers' markets can serve as "community spaces" and raises questions about the staffing and organizational models that might best encourage this potential. Whether alongside or in place of making a "direct connection between consumer and the people who grow their food" (CDC 2011: 21), mobile markets might productively focus on facilitating connections between community members. One aspect of such connections is built into the structure of the SMFM, where the primary farm providing produce at the SMFM does not do direct sales; rather the market manager, who is a resident of the Mystic and appears to be a trusted confidant and important source of information for shoppers, is responsible for sales, while other sales are conducted by local youth. Additionally, a wide variety of health, arts, and educational organizations host booths during the season. This highlights the multiple kinds of information and resources that can be shared – not only between vendors and shoppers, but also among community members – at farmers' markets. Indeed, we need to know more about the economic, social, and health benefits of conversations and connections among all market participants.

We would especially encourage research on how recent immigrant groups use farmers' markets. Immigrants may have more recent experiences with markets as the center of local communities, as noted by the Food Dignity Project, "[M]any people come to US cities from places where open-air markets were the norm ..." (Daftary-Steele 2014: 3). Given that acculturation to American dietary habits may be one mechanism by which successive generations experience worsening health status (Abraido-Lanza, Chao and Florez 2005), supporting immigrants' preferences for culturally relevant fruit and vegetables may prove to be a powerful public health intervention. It appears that we have much to learn from recent immigrants regarding how to organize markets that meet a variety of health and social objectives.

More broadly, the SMFM offers an interesting counter-example in regard to many of the stereotypes and associated critiques of farmers' markets in regard to food justice. While nationally, the average farmers' market customer may be white, middle to upper class, and well educated, there is clearly significant demand for fresh produce among the low-income and immigrant shoppers of the SMFM.

Critics of farmers markets contend that claims about the value of consumer education and relationship building between customers and farmers represent a "white imaginary" that hearkens back to a romanticized pastoral vision of farming (Alkon and McCullen 2010). However, this white imaginary is clearly upended at Somerville markets where local youth, recent immigrants and farmers of diverse racial and ethnic backgrounds will be selling callaloo and calabash – and a variety of other goods – to low-income and immigrant shoppers (see also Daftary-Steele 2014; Suarez-Balcazar, et al. 2006). The possibility of making space at the markets available to urban growers might also support the goal of making connections between the people growing food and the people purchasing (and eating) it. And, while the SMFM has met with challenges in bringing food to low-income and immigrant communities that is culturally appropriate or desirable, it also has demonstrated that markets can evolve in response to community feedback.

That said, the meaning of "local" food – and the strong desire for tropical fruits among patrons of the SMFM – highlights ongoing tensions between the goals of sustainability and food sovereignty and cultural appropriateness. Ideally, seeing the SMFM respond to their requests will lead to other forms of engagement and empowerment among Somerville's most recent residents. Allowing urban farmers to sell at the markets might further support the emergence of markets as a site of transformative political engagement, by bringing neighbors into explicit conversation with each other about food production, food access, and health in the City.

We recognize that as a case study in a single city, our findings are neither definitive nor generalizable. Rather, we hope that they will serve as a jumping off point for further analyses. Nonetheless, we believe that this mixed-methods approach to studying a mobile market identifies important opportunities for collaboration and conversation among stakeholders committed to improving food access and addressing issues of food justice. Likewise, it highlights the importance of attending the foodways and preferences of members of the city's low-income and immigrant communities as an essential aspect of these efforts.

Acknowledgements

We are grateful for the support of David Hudson, formerly the Director of Shape Up Somerville, and Kawsar Jahan, the SMFM manager. We thank the Groundwork Somerville Green Team for their enthusiastic and excellent research assistance at the Market, and their careful collaborative tabulation of the dot survey data. We appreciate the insightful feedback we received at the Feeding Cities Workshop at Northeastern University in March, 2015; thanks especially to Carole Biewener for her analysis of our work.

Notes

1 Available online at www.fns.usda.gov/pressrelease/2015/027315 (accessed September 7, 2016).
2 The USDA's report to Congress is available at www.ers.usda.gov/media/242675/ap036_1_.pdf (accessed October 12, 2014).

3 Available online at www.ams.usda.gov/AMSv1.0/ams.fetchTemplateData.do?template =TemplateSandleftNav=WholesaleandFarmersMarketsandpage=WF (accessed October 12, 2014).
4 Available online at www.bostonglobe.com/lifestyle/food-dining/2013/08/06/bay-state-ranks-number-farmers-markets/JcwN2d55s6D3UuaQlecojJ/story.html (accessed October 12, 2014).
5 Available online at www.usda.gov/wps/portal/usda/usdahome?contentid=2012/08/0262.xml (accessed October 12, 2014).
6 Available online at www.groundworksomerville.org/programs/green-jobs/green-team/ (accessed January 14, 2016).
7 Unfortunately, our data collection dates for October and November were cancelled due to inclement weather. However, by then, the diminishing number of responses gathered on each successive day made clear that we had surveyed a preponderance of the SMFM customers.
8 Available online at http://quickfacts.census.gov/qfd/states/25/2562535.html (accessed February 1, 2015). For a history of settlement and population trends, see www.somervillema.gov/sites/default/files/CompPLan/Population%20Trends%20Report%205-19_Final1.pdf (accessed October 12, 2014).
9 The Liaison Interpreter Program of Somerville (LIPS) is a program for youth organized by the Welcome Project. LIPS "provides opportunities for bilingual high school students to learn language interpretation skills and to practice those skills at community meetings and events throughout the city." Available online at www.welcomeproject.org/content/liaison-interpreters-program-somerville-lips (accessed February 25, 2015).
10 See for example, URL: http://nesfp.org/foodaccess and https://foodinthehood.wordpress.com/2012/05/02/farm-share-registration-for-bowdoin-geneva-families-now-open/ (both accessed October 3, 2015).

References

Abraido-Lanza, A., Chao, M., and Florez, K. 2005. "Do health behaviors decline with greater acculturation?: Implications for the Latino mortality paradox." *Social Science and Medicine* 61: 1243–1255.
Abusabha, R., Namjoshi, D., and Klen, A. 2011. "Increasing access and affordability of produce improves perceived consumption of vegetables in low-income seniors." *Journal of the American Dietetic Association* 111 (10): 1549–1555.
Alkon, A., and McCullen, C. 2010. "Whiteness and farmers markets: Performances, perpetuations contestations?" *Antipode* 43 (4): 937–959.
Alkon, A., and Agyeman, J. 2011. *Cultivating Food Justice: Race, Class, and Sustainability.* Cambridge, MA: MIT University Press.
Alkon, A., and Mares, T. 2012. "Food sovereignty in US food movements: Radical visions and neoliberal constraints." *Agriculture and Human Values* 29 (3): 347–359.
Alkon, A., Block, D., Moore, K., Gillis, C., DiNuccio, N., and Chavez, N. "Foodways of the urban poor." *Geoforum* 48: 126–135.
Baronberg, S., Dunn, L., Nonas, C., Dannefer, R., and Sacks, R. 2013. "The impact of New York City's Health Bucks Program on electronic benefit transfer spending at farmers markets, 2006–2009." *Preventing Chronic Disease* 10: 130113.
Block, J., Scribner R., and De Salvo, K. 2004. "Fast food, race/ethnicity, and income: A geographic analysis." *American Journal of Preventive Medicine* 27 (3): 211–217.
Brown, A. 2002. "Farmers' market research 1940–2000: An inventory and review." *American Journal of Alternative Agriculture* 17 (4): 167–176.

Cannuscio, C., Weiss, E., and Asch, D. 2010. "The contribution of urban foodways to health disparities." *Journal of Urban Health* 87 (3): 381–393.

Caspi C., Kawachi, I., Subramanian, S.V., Adamkiewicz, G., and Sorensen, G. 2012a. "The relationship between diet and perceived and objective access to supermarkets among low-income housing residents." *Social Science and Medicine* 75: 1254–1262.

Caspi, C., Sorensen, G., Subramanian, S.V., and Kawachi, I. 2012b. "The local food environment and diet: A systematic review." *Health and Place* 18 (5): 1172–1187.

Centers for Disease Prevention and Control. 2011. *The CDC Guide to Increase the Consumption of Fruits and Vegetables*. Available online at www.cdc.gov/obesity/downloads/FandV2011WEBTAG508.pdf (accessed February 6, 2015).

Charmaz, K. 2006. *Constructing Grounded Theory: A Practical Guide through Qualitative Analysis*. Thousand Oaks, CA: SAGE.

Cummins, S., Flint, E., and Matthews, S. 2014. "New neighborhood grocery store increased awareness of food access but did not alter dietary habits or obesity." *Health Affairs* 32 (2): 283–291.

Daftary-Steel, S. 2014. *Building a Great Farmers' Market*. Food Dignity Brief #2. Available online at http://fooddignity.org/wp/wp-content/uploads/2014/12/Practical guide-Communitybasedfarmersmarkets-v5_reduced-size.pdf (accessed May 14, 2015).

Elbel, B., Moran, A., Dixon, L.B., Kiszko, K., Cantor, J., Abrams, C., and Mijanovich, T. 2015. "Assessment of a government-subsidized supermarket in a high-need area on household food availability and children's dietary intakes." *Public Health Nutrition* 26: 1–10.

Emerson, R., Fretz, R., and Shaw, L. 1995. *Writing Ethnographic Fieldnotes*. Chicago: University of Chicago Press.

Evans, A., Jennings, R., Smiley, A.W., Medina, J.L., Sharma, S.V., Rutledge, R., Stigler, M.H., and Hoelscher, D.M. 2012. "Introduction of farm stands in low-income communities increases fruit and vegetable among community residents." *Health and Place* 18 (5): 1137–1143.

Freedman, D.A., Mattison-Faye, A., Alia, K., Guest, M.A., and Hébert, J.R.. 2014. "Comparing farmers' market revenue trends before and after the implementation of a monetary incentive for recipients of food assistance." *Preventing Chronic Disease* 11: 130347.

Freudenberg, N., and Galea, S. 2008. "Cities of consumption: The impact of corporate practices on the health of urban populations." *Journal of Urban Health* 85 (4): 462–471.

Guthman, J. 2008. "Bringing good food to others: Investigating the subjects of alternative food institutions." *Cultural Geographies* 15 (4): 387–397.

Holben, D. 2011. "Farmers' markets: Fertile ground for optimizing health." *Journal of the American Dietetic Association*, Commentary, 364–365.

Kato, Y., and McKinney, L. 2014. "Bringing food desert residents to an alternative food market: A semi-experimental study of impediments to food access." *Agriculture and Human Values* [published online: DOI 10.1007/s10460-014-9541-3].

Larsen, K., and Gilliland, J. 2009. "A farmers' market in a food desert: Evaluating impact on the price and availability of healthy food." *Health and Place* 15: 1158–1162.

Latham, J., and Moffat, T. 2007. "Determinants of variation in food cost and availability in two socioeconomically contrasting neighbourhoods of Hamilton, Ontario, Canada." *Health and Place* 13: 273–287.

LeDoux, T., and Vojnovic, I. 2013. "Going outside the neighborhood: The shopping patterns and adaptations of disadvantaged consumers living in the lower eastside neighborhoods of Detroit, Michigan." *Health and Place* 19: 1–14.

Lev, L., Brewer, L., and Stephenson, G. 2008. *Tools for Rapid Market Assessments*. Special Report 1088-E; Oregon Small Farms Technical Report No. 6. Oregon State University Extension Service.

Lewis, C., and Zollinger, T. 2012. *Garden on the Go demonstration study report*. Indiana University Health. Available online at https://iuhealth.org/images/uploads/Final_Report_Garden_on_the_Go_Demonstration_Study.pdf (accessed February 18, 2015).

Lyson, M. 2014. "The class politics of alternative food: Informing public health policy and remedying health inequality." *Sociology Compass* 8/10: 1216–1228.

McCormack, L., Laska, M.N., Larson, N.I., and Story, M. 2010. "Review of the nutritional implications of farmers' markets and community gardens: A call for evaluation and research efforts." *Journal of the American Dietetic Association* 110 (3): 399–408.

Moore, L., and Diez Roux, A. 2006. "Associations of neighborhood characteristics with the location and type of food stores." *American Journal Public Health* 96 (2): 325–331.

Morland, K., and Filomena, S. 2007. "Disparities in the availability of fruits and vegetables between racially segregated urban neighbourhoods." *Public Health Nutrition* 10 (12): 1481–1489.

Morland, K., and Evenson, K. 2009. "Obesity prevalence and the local food environment." *Health and Place* 15: 491–495.

Morland, K., Wing, S., Diez Roux, A., and Poole, C. 2002. "Neighborhood characteristics associated with the location of food stores and food service places." *American Journal of Preventive Medicine* 22(1): 23–29.

Morland, K., Diez Roux, A., and Wing, S. 2006. "Supermarkets, other food stores, and obesity: The atherosclerosis risk in communities study." *American Journal of Preventive Medicine* 30 (4): 333–339.

Ostrander, S. 2013. *Citizenship and Governance in a Changing City: Somerville, MA*. Philadelphia: Temple University Press.

Philadelphia Greensgrow Project (2012). *Using Mobile Markets to Provide Healthy Food Retail Outlets in Food Deserts and Low-Income Areas of Camden City, New Jersey*. Philadelphia: Greensgrow.

Powell, L., Slater, S., Mirtcheva, D., Bao, Y., and Chaloupka, F.J. 2007. "Food store availability and neighborhood characteristics in the United States." *Preventive Medicine* 44: 189–195.

Ruelas, V., Iverson, E., Kiekel, P., and Peters, A. 2012. "The role of farmers' markets in two low income, urban communities." *Journal of Community Health* 37: 554–562.

Slocum, R. 2007. "Whiteness, space, and alternative food practice." *Geoforum* 38 (3): 520–533.

Suarez-Balcazar, Y., Martinez, L.I., Cox, G., and Jayraj, A. 2006. "African Americans' views of access to healthy foods: What a farmers' market provides." *Journal of Extension* 44 (2). Available online at http://www.joe.org/joe/2006april/a2p.shtml (accessed February 12, 2015).

Tester, J., Yen, I., and Laraia, B. 2012. "Using mobile fruit market vendors to increase access to fresh fruit and vegetables for school children." *Preventing Chronic Disease*. Available online at http://www.cdc.gov/pcd/issues/2012/11_0222.htm (accessed February 18, 2015).

Union Square Main Streets (USMS). 2010. *Union Square Farmers' Market Report*. Somerville, MA.

Walker, R., Keane, C., and Burke, J. 2010. "Disparities and access to health food in the United States: A review of food deserts literature." *Health and Place* 16: 876–884.

Widener, M., Metcalf, S., and Bar-Yam, Y. 2012. "Developing a mobile produce distribution system for low-income urban residents in food deserts." *Journal of Urban Health* 89 (5): 733–745.

Young, C,. Aquilante, J.L., Solomon, S., Colby, L., Kawinzi, M.A., Uy, N., and Mallya, G. 2013. "Improving fruit and vegetable consumption among low-income customers at farmers markets: Philly Food Bucks, Philadelphia, Pennsylvania." *Preventing Chronic Disease* 10: 120356.

Zenk, S., Schulz, A.J., Israel, B.A., James, S.A., Bao, S., and Wilson, M.L. 2005. "Neighbourhood racial composition, neighborhood poverty, and the spatial accessibility of supermarkets in metropolitan Detroit." *American Journal of Public Health* 95: 660–667.

Zepeda, L. 2009. "Which little piggy goes to market? Characteristics of US farmers' market shoppers." *International Journal of Consumer Studies* 33 (3): 250–257.

Zepeda, L., Reznickova, A., and Lohr, L. 2014. "Overcoming challenges to effectiveness of mobile markets in US food deserts." *Appetite* 79: 58–67.

6   Farm to home

Senior Farmers' Market Nutrition Program access and fresh fruit and vegetable home delivery for homebound older adults

Mehreen Ismail and Cara Cuite

For aging adults, eating adequate amounts of fruits and vegetables may help prevent or manage chronic disease and promote health and quality of life (Institute of Medicine 2012; Van Duyn and Pivonka 2000). Yet some seniors, particularly those who are homebound, face many barriers to eating fruit and vegetables. These include problems of physical access, as those with limited mobility may have difficulty getting to a store or market, and cost, as lower income seniors may not be able to afford fresh fruits and vegetables.

The project described here capitalizes on synergies between two federal programs that are designed to improve the diets and health of seniors. One is the Senior Farmers' Market Nutrition Program (SFMNP), which was designed to assist low-income seniors in affording fresh fruit and vegetables. The SFMNP increases affordability of fresh fruit and vegetables sold in farmers' markets, at roadside stands, and through community supported agriculture (CSA) programs (USDA Food and Nutrition Service 2014). The program provides $20 – $50 worth of vouchers to income-eligible applicants, depending on state of residence, distributing approximately $20.5 million in benefits in 2014 (USDA Food and Nutrition Service 2015a). The other program, administered through Title IIIC of the Older Americans Act (OAA), provides home-delivered meals, commonly referred to as "meals on wheels" (U.S. DHHS Administration for Community Living n.d.) This program targets homebound seniors. In 2015, over $216 million was appropriated for home-delivered meals in the form of grants to states and community programs on aging (Napili and Collelo 2015). Agencies that deliver meals raise many more dollars, either through client donations or other fundraising efforts (Meals on Wheels America 2015).

This chapter describes a small intervention study in which a subset of home-delivered meal program clients also were enrolled in the SFMNP, and the home-delivered meal program infrastructure was used to provide home delivery of fresh fruits and vegetables purchased partially with SFMNP funds. We describe the programs and partners involved, project logistics, and findings from the intervention evaluation. We conclude with a discussion of limitations and lessons learned.

Senior Farmers' Market Nutrition Program

The SFMNP provides coupons for low-income seniors to use for purchasing fresh fruits and vegetables at direct-to-consumer operations, including farmers' markets. The program is part of a suite of federal nutrition assistance programs targeted toward older adults (Gergerich, Shobe, and Christy 2015). SFMNP is unique in its focus on increasing affordability specifically for fresh, locally grown fruits and vegetables (USDA Food and Nutrition Service 2014; Gergerich et al. 2015).

The United States Department of Agriculture (USDA) funds and regulates SFMNP, which is currently administered through 52 state agencies and federally recognized Indian tribal governments (USDA Food and Nutrition Service 2014). Following a trial period with Senior Farmers' Market Nutrition Pilot Program in 2001, the Farm Security and Rural Investment Act of 2002 (otherwise known as the "Farm Bill") expanded the program and provided $80 million in funding for fiscal years (FY) 2002–2007. The purpose of the SFMNP is to increase the resources with which low-income older adults could purchase locally grown fruits, vegetables, and herbs. Through augmented consumer demand, another program aim was to assist in development and expansion of farmers' markets, roadside stands, and community CSA programs. While the 2002 law established temporary competitive funding (USDA Food and Nutrition Service 2006), the SFMNP was made permanent in 2007 and maintained goals consistent with those from previous legislation (USDA Food and Nutrition Service 2007). In FY 2014, program administrators served over 787,000 low-income seniors (USDA Food and Nutrition Service 2015a).

A broad set of criteria governs who may participate in SFMNP and where and when benefits may be used. Only those who are aged 60 years or older and who have income at or below 185 percent of the Federal Poverty Level may participate. Seniors must apply for the program every year. If approved, participants receive $20 – $50 worth of coupons that can be redeemed at farmers' markets, roadside stands, and CSA programs. Given that benefit redemption is restricted to specific direct-to-consumer operations, SFMNP participants may have a limited time frame during which benefits can be used (USDA Food and Nutrition Service 2014). For example, in New Jersey, approved SFMNP participants are granted four $5 coupons, which must be used between June and November during a given year (State of NJ Department of Health 2015).

To date there are few academic evaluations of the SFMNP or other similar state-level programs (McCormack et al. 2010). Some of the earliest evaluations come from Massachusetts and South Carolina. Researchers in both states found that sizable proportions of seniors who received coupons and participated in the evaluation studies had intentions either to continue shopping at farmers' markets or to continue buying produce, even after exhausting the value of their coupons (Webber, Balsam, and Oehlke 1995; Kunkel, Luccia, and Moore 2003). Neither evaluation study included direct measures of fruit and vegetable consumption. However, evaluators in Massachusetts found that survey respondents spent an additional $5.60 on average on produce (Webber et al. 1995), suggesting that the quantity purchased was more than what could have been obtained using coupons alone. Three out of five survey respondents in South Carolina reported that having coupons changed the way they ate (Kunkel et al. 2003). These evaluations convey the benefits of coupons that subsidize fruit and vegetable purchases, at least for low-income older adults who are mobile and able to visit farmers' markets.

Two projects connecting homebound seniors with SFMNP also have been evaluated. By enlisting support from local farmers with USDA and SFMNP funding and by partnering with existing home-delivered meal programs, projects in Seattle, Washington and northeast Georgia offered home deliveries of fresh fruit and vegetables to home-delivered meal program clients. Evaluators found high program satisfaction, increased fruit and vegetable consumption, and high coupon redemption rates (Johnson et al. 2004; Sinnett et al. 2009). The intervention described in this chapter builds on the work done in Washington and Georgia, applying a similar model to serve home-delivered meal program clients in New Brunswick, New Jersey.

Meals on Wheels of Greater New Brunswick

Under Title IIIC of the Older Americans Act, the federal government funds home-delivered meal programs to provide food and social contact for homebound seniors. These programs provide support for seniors to age in place and live independently. Homebound seniors may take advantage of such services if they have limited ability to shop for and to prepare meals (Meals on Wheels America 2015).

In Middlesex County, New Jersey, the Office of Aging and Disabled Services administers the SFMNP and runs a home-delivered meal program for residents throughout the County, including the city of New Brunswick. In addition to this county program, private non-profit services are available through Meals on Wheels of Greater New Brunswick (MOWGNB), which since 1973 has been delivering meals to homebound seniors in the Greater New Brunswick area, including the neighboring borough of Highland Park. At the time of the intervention, MOWGNB was serving 65 seniors in the geographic areas depicted in Figure 6.1. Volunteers deliver one hot and one cold meal to each client every weekday. Meals are funded through private donations and federal reimbursements (Meals on Wheels in Greater New Brunswick n.d.). Both locally and nationally, home-delivered meal programs like MOWGNB provide clients with a substantial proportion of their dietary intake and fill a critical gap for those who are unable to shop independently at a grocery store or farmers' market (Meals on Wheels America 2015).

MOWGNB works with a nutritionist to ensure that meals are nutritionally appropriate. Typically, meals include fresh fruit, fruit juice, and cooked vegetables. Although fruits and vegetables are offered, the quantities provided may not satisfy recommendations for daily servings of fruits and vegetables. Additionally, since breakfast and weekend meals are not delivered (Meals on Wheels in Greater New Brunswick n.d.), there is no guarantee that clients are able to meet daily fruit and

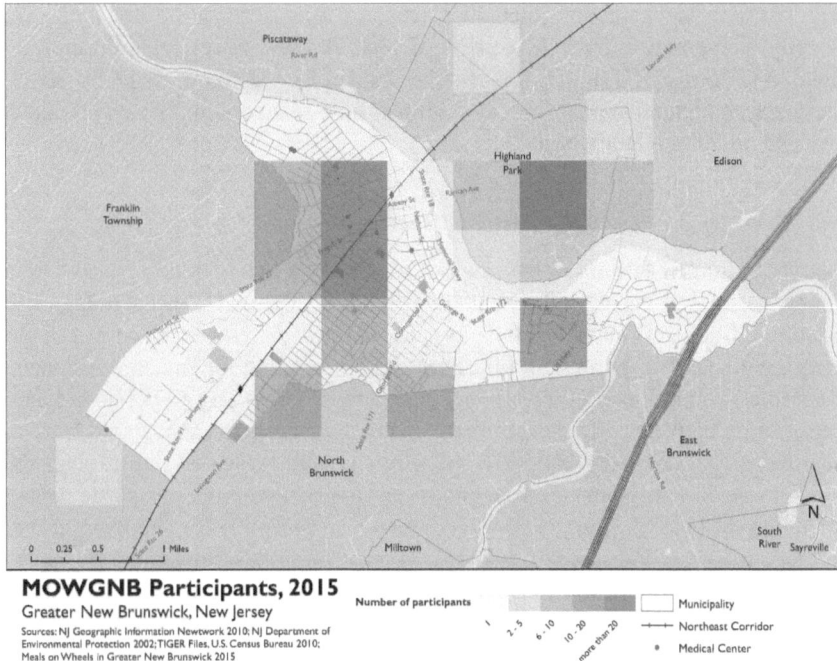

MOWGNB Participants, 2015
Greater New Brunswick, New Jersey

Sources: NJ Geographic Information Newtwork 2010; NJ Department of
Environmental Protection 2002; TIGER Files, U.S. Census Bureau 2010;
Meals on Wheels in Greater New Brunswick 2015

Figure 6.1   Distribution and density of Meals on Wheels of Greater New Brunswick
participants

vegetable recommendations. Indeed, there is evidence suggesting that some home-
delivered meal program clients may not have much additional food in their homes.
Specifically, food inventory audits considering a multi-state sample of 750
households with home-delivered meal program clients found many to have little to
no available fresh food, much less fresh fruits and vegetables (Hallman et al., in
preparation). Given this finding, the potential gap that MOWGNB was leaving
unfilled, and its existing relationship with Rutgers University-led research projects
(e.g., Cuite, Dahwan, and Fitz 2013), the intervention sought to increase household
availability of fresh fruits and vegetables for greater New Brunswick's homebound
seniors, who otherwise may not be able to reach a grocery store or farmers' market.

New Brunswick in context

In the few years preceding the intervention, New Brunswick became an incubator
for activity around its local food system (New Brunswick Community Food
Alliance 2014), making it a notable case study site. The city, located in central
New Jersey, was home to approximately 57,000 residents in 2014. New Brunswick
is younger and poorer relative to the state overall. In 2010, 13.5 percent of New
Jersey's population was comprised of people aged 65 years or older, while just 5
percent of New Brunswick's population was part of this age group. Between 2009

and 2013, it was estimated that 10 percent of New Jerseyans were living in poverty, compared to over 33 percent of New Brunswick residents during the same time period (U.S. Census Bureau 2015). Low-income residents are a particular target audience for the multiple food-related initiatives that have cropped up in New Brunswick.

New Brunswick Community Farmers' Market

One such initiative is the New Brunswick Community Farmers' Market (NBCFM), which began serving the city in 2009 (Biemiller 2009). Unlike a previously established farmers' market in the city, the NBCFM places greater emphasis on carrying ethnically appropriate offerings and on reaching low-income residents (Biemiller 2009; Lawson, Fitzgerald, and Drake 2016). As a public–private partnership between city government, a public land-grant university, and a pharmaceutical company, the NBCFM works toward the latter aim through its Market Bucks program. Federal nutrition assistance program participants, including those taking part in SFMNP, receive an incentive for shopping at the farmers' market (Cuite and Dixon 2015). At the time of the intervention, for every $5 of federal nutrition assistance program benefits spent, shoppers received an additional $2 to spend at the NBCFM. The incentive program illustrates the NBCFM's commitment to ensuring affordable access to fresh, locally grown fruits and vegetables for New Brunswick residents (Cuite and Dixon 2015). Despite this commitment, there was reason to believe that the NBCFM was not reaching *all* city residents, particularly those who are homebound. Hence the rationale for the pilot intervention described next.

Intervention

A fresh fruit and vegetable home delivery intervention was launched in summer 2014 to address potential lack of availability, and for some, affordability, of these foods among MOWGNB clients. The intervention included two components and involved multiple stakeholders.

SFMNP in-home application assistance

The first intervention component occurred before home deliveries could begin. It involved laying the groundwork for the remainder of the intervention by identifying partners and funding sources. The MOWGNB and NBCFM were early partners, each committing to distinct features of the home delivery intervention component. The NBCFM also committed to funding a portion of fruit and vegetable costs. The value of this contribution filled in gaps that the other main funding source could not cover.

Given that some MOWGNB clients were of low income, the SFMNP was recognized as a partial funding stream. However, SFMNP enrollment in the Greater New Brunswick area occurs only in-person at a rotating list of senior centers and senior housing buildings (L. Higgins, personal communication, May 21, 2014). Connecting homebound MOWGNB clients, who could not necessarily access these locations, to the federal program emerged as a challenge. By entering into discussions with the Middlesex County Office of Aging and Disabled Services, an SFMNP-administering agency, the authors gained permission to conduct in-home SFMNP application assistance. Figure 6.2 describes the procedures followed to enroll MOWGNB clients into the program. Clients who successfully enrolled in the SFMNP through this process were offered the option to use their SFMNP coupons independent of the intervention; however, no clients pursued this option.

When considering the SFMNP enrollment process undertaken, it is important to note that only a fraction of MOWGNB clients were eligible for the program to begin with. Eligibility for SFMNP is largely based on age and income (USDA Food and Nutrition Service 2014), and as such does not entirely overlap with eligibility for home-delivered meals funded through Title IIIC of the OAA. The

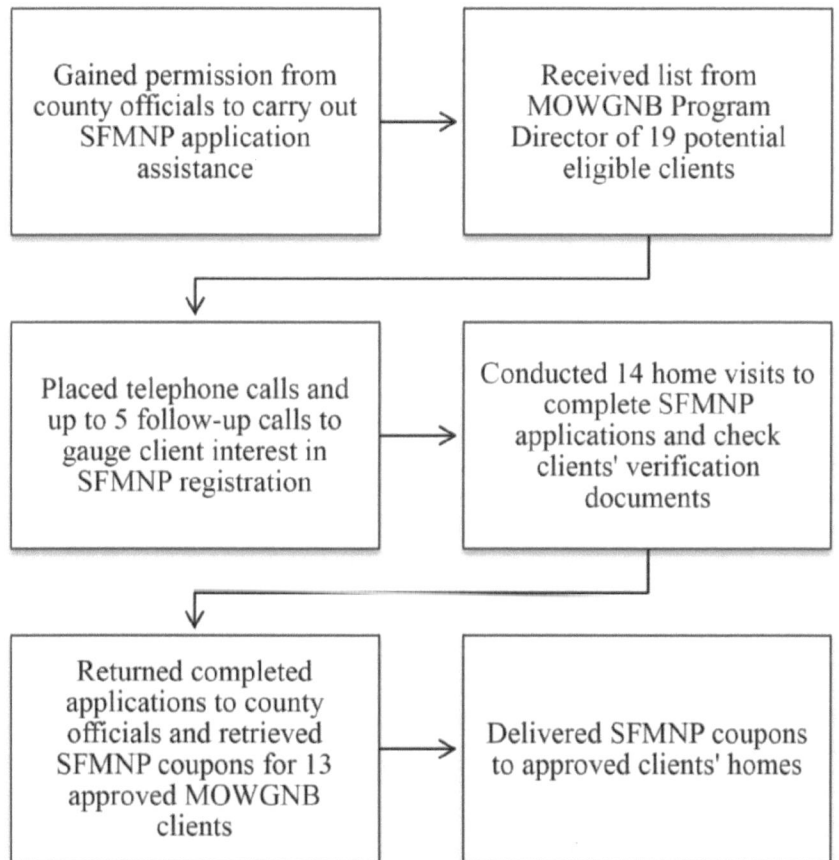

Figure 6.2   SFMNP in-home application assistance process

latter federal program uses age and physical functioning impairments, not age and income, as its guiding criteria (DHHS Administration for Community Living n.d.). Therefore, higher income MOWGNB clients were ineligible for SFMNP and were not included in the application assistance effort.

As noted, the NBCFM's funding commitment covered purchasing costs that SFMNP could not, either due to client ineligibility or disinterest. The market's sizable contribution allowed all non-SFMNP participating clients to receive home deliveries at no cost. To ensure that all MOWGNB clients received an equitable share of fresh fruits and vegetables, and to keep costs down, offerings were capped at what could be purchased with SFMNP coupons. Annual SFMNP allotments in New Jersey include four $5-coupons per participant. With the NBCFM's Market Bucks program, an additional $2 for every $5 of SFMNP benefits could be leveraged. In practice, this meant delivering $7 worth of fresh fruits and vegetables per client per four home deliveries, or $28 worth overall.

Fresh fruit and vegetable home deliveries

The second component of the intervention entailed working out home delivery logistics and implementing home deliveries. Promotion about this component occurred over the telephone and through flyers accompanying clients' regular home-delivered meals. Clients were informed of intervention dates; four bi-weekly home deliveries occurred between late June and early August. Additionally, clients were informed of their ability to withdraw from the intervention at any time.

Prior to each of the four home deliveries, the authors consulted with the NBCFM market manager to determine home delivery offerings. As part of its typical services, MOWGNB provides all clients with the same hot and cold meals. To remain consistent, all clients received identical types and quantities of fresh fruits and vegetables throughout the intervention. This meant that only fruits and vegetables that the participating farmer could obtain in sufficient quantities could be included in the produce bags.

Based on advice from a researcher who implemented a similar project in Washington State (M. Podrabsky, personal communication, May 22, 2014), the authors and the market manager placed emphasis on selecting fresh fruit for the home deliveries. Choosing fresh fruits and vegetables that required minimal processing by clients was also a priority. Further limiting the selection were restrictions on what could be purchased using SFMNP benefits. Given SFMNP's priority to promote local agriculture, program benefits can be redeemed only for fresh fruits, vegetables, and herbs grown within a given state (USDA Food and Nutrition Service 2014). Although locally grown and produced items are central to the NBCFM, its vendors are also permitted to carry items imported into New Jersey. Since some of these imported goods, like bananas, are easy to consume, they were included in the home deliveries. To comply with SFMNP requirements, however, only $2 per client per home delivery were allotted for such "non-conforming" items, corresponding to the value of the Market Bucks incentive.

Once the market manager and vendor finalized contents to be included, the fresh fruits and vegetables could be prepared for home delivery. The NBCFM's market manager, volunteers, and this chapter's two authors packed individual bags for each client on afternoons before intervention days. Bags were stored in a commercial refrigerator located in the kitchen where clients' meals were prepared. On the morning of deliveries, the authors placed nutrition education materials, vegetable preparation tips, and feedback forms inside the bags. Bags designated for the 13 SFMNP participants were specially labeled to alert MOWGNB volunteers about retrieving SFMNP coupons from those individuals.

MOWGNB volunteers played a key role in the intervention's second component. On intervention days, the authors briefed volunteers about the intervention verbally and with a one-page handout. The authors also instructed volunteers to collect SFMNP coupons and to return them to the MOWGNB office. As per MOWGNB protocol, any undeliverable meals were to be returned with their accompanying fresh fruit and vegetable bags as well. This applied if clients failed to notify the MOWGNB program director about their absence at time of delivery. Although delivering bags of fresh fruits and vegetables along with clients' regular home-delivered meals presented volunteers with an additional responsibility, volunteers anecdotally gave positive feedback about the intervention. Having volunteer buy-in facilitated intervention implementation and allowed fresh fruit and vegetable home deliveries to occur within the context of an established home-delivered meal program.

Following each home delivery, the authors completed post-delivery tasks at the MOWGNB office and at the NBCFM. Any undeliverable bags were distributed to kitchen or MOWGNB staff. One of the authors also collected returned feedback forms and SFMNP coupons. Coupons were given to the SFMNP-authorized vendor, who supplied all of the fresh fruits and vegetables for the intervention. The NBCFM market manager then paid the vendor the balance depending on how many SFMNP coupons had been returned. Paying the vendor represented the final step of intervention implementation and bridged both intervention components.

Evaluation insights

The authors engaged in a brief evaluation of the intervention to understand its reach, implementation, and effectiveness. This involved tracking a series of measures throughout the intervention and interviewing MOWGNB clients after the home delivery component ended.

Reach and implementation: methods and findings

One measure that most directly involved clients included the number of fresh fruit and vegetable bags delivered. Over four home deliveries, MOWGNB volunteers delivered 214 bags of fresh fruits and vegetables. If home deliveries had reached all 64 MOWGNB clients on all intervention days, volunteers would have delivered 256 bags. The actual number of bags delivered was approximately 17 percent lower than this projected figure, primarily due to clients being absent from their homes on intervention days.

Another measure directly involving clients was the number of SFMNP coupons redeemed. The subset of clients participating in the federal program redeemed 50 coupons over the course of the intervention. Since 13 MOWGNB clients received four SFMNP coupons each, a total of 52 coupons could have been redeemed. Two clients either lost or misplaced the last coupon they had received, yielding a 96 percent redemption rate. Compared to the 90 percent redemption rate for the county overall (L. Higgins, personal communication, May 21, 2014), the intervention performed slightly better, albeit accounting for a much smaller number of SFMNP participants.

Other aspects of the intervention including costs were tracked, but occurred behind the scenes. The value of redeemed SFMNP coupons amounted to $250; NBCFM had to contribute $1,326 to cover remaining fruit and vegetable purchasing costs. Of this contribution, over one in four dollars were sourced from Market Bucks matching funds. Knowing that some MOWGNB clients would be absent on intervention days, the NBCFM market manager placed orders to fill just 60 fresh fruit and vegetable bags per home delivery. Given this figure and the projection that each bag would be worth $7, fresh fruit and vegetable purchasing costs should have totaled $1,680. Actual costs were $104 under this budget. Since the vendor sold quantities in bulk, the market manager was able to negotiate lower price points, resulting in savings.

Since personnel and volunteers involved in the intervention were not compensated, time devoted to implementation was another appropriate measure to track. Accounting for all home deliveries and for multiple volunteers, the first and second intervention components required approximately 36 and 26 hours to complete, respectively. This does not, however, account for time needed to deliver fresh fruit and vegetable bags; there was no evidence to suggest that MOWGNB volunteers required extra time to complete home deliveries. The first component's steps, as described in Figure 6.2, took more time to complete yet yielded only $250 in redeemed SFMNP benefits. Given the small fraction of funding obtained, it was ultimately not cost effective to register MOWGNB clients for the federal program.

Effectiveness: methods

In addition to tracking measures related to intervention reach and implementation, the authors interviewed MOWGNB clients about their intervention experiences. Clients were eligible for an interview if they met all of the following criteria:

- Still receiving MOWGNB services at the time of interviewee recruitment.
- Not absent from home due to medical or personal reasons during interviewee recruitment.
- English-speaking.
- Not severely cognitive impaired.
- Received at least one fresh fruit and vegetable home delivery.

Recruitment for a convenience sample of interviewees took place over the telephone. Each potential interviewee received up to three initial or follow-up telephone calls. Out of a pool of 48 clients, 17 individuals agreed to complete a recorded interview either over the telephone or in person.

Interview questions were similar to those used for an evaluation study conducted in Seattle, Washington (Smith et al. 2004). Topics included past farmers' market exposure and perceptions of the fresh fruit and vegetable home delivery intervention. An adapted screener from the Behavioral Risk Factor Surveillance System (BRFSS) was used to quantify fruit and vegetable intake. Although the screener typically asks for respondents to recall intake from the past month (Centers for Disease Control and Prevention 2012), the authors modified the recall period to reflect the past week to reduce cognitive difficulty. While all interviewees were questioned about their familiarity with the SFMNP, only those involved in the first intervention component were asked about their in-home application assistance experience. To cover these topics, interviews lasted between 10 and 25 minutes. Rutgers University Institutional Review Board approved all interview procedures.

Since the interview protocol included both open- and closed-ended questions, the author responsible for analysis took two approaches to summarizing responses. Closed-ended responses were coded, whereas open-ended responses were transcribed. Each interview recording was reviewed at least twice to accomplish these tasks. Wherever possible, simple descriptive statistics were calculated. Transcripts were reviewed to identify themes.

Table 6.1 describes demographic characteristics of the interview sample and of all MOWGNB clients receiving services two weeks post-intervention. The MOWGNB program director furnished administrative records containing data on all clients. Although race/ethnicity information was captured in both the interviews and administrative records, data are not presented since response options did not match. Qualitatively, it appears that the interview sample was not representative of MOWGNB clients overall, especially in terms of poverty level. Therefore the following findings should be interpreted without necessarily generalizing to clients who participated in the intervention but not in an interview.

Table 6.1 Demographic characteristics of interviewees relative to all MOWGNB clients

	All MOWGNB clients n = 63	Interview sample n = 17
Female (%)	64%	59%
Age (median, years)	76	72
Poverty (% at or below federal poverty level)	25	46

n = 16
b n = 13

Farmers' market patronage

Since the intervention forged a connection between the NBCFM and MOWGNB clients' homes, understanding whether interviewees were familiar with farmers' markets was of interest. Past farmers' market patronage was a common experience; over 80 percent of interviewees stated they had been to this type of direct-to-consumer operation prior to the intervention. Of these respondents, one in three volunteered information about a present inability to shop at farmers' markets. Some reasons included no longer being the primary food shopper or being physically impaired. For example, one interviewee whose husband received MOWGNB services shared, "We are kind of incapacitated ... so we rarely travel far from the house." Another client mentioned how NBCFM was right around the corner from her home; however, due to her limited mobility, she was not able to access the farmers' market until the intervention began. Similar comments from other interviewees indicated that the intervention reconnected homebound seniors to a type of retail outlet, which, in the past, had been more accessible.

SFMNP awareness and participation

Although the SFMNP increases farmers' market affordability, the program, like farmers' markets themselves, may be inaccessible for homebound older adults. Despite its potential inaccessibility, interviews sought to determine levels of SFMNP awareness. Interviewees were not necessarily income-eligible for the program; however, since income information was not collected until the end of the interview, all interviewees were asked about the program. Prior to the intervention, only four out of 17 interviewees had heard of the SFMNP when asked about it by name.

At least eight interviewees were eligible for the program, since they had participated in the first intervention component. Of these interviewees, two commented on the convenience of in-home application assistance. One of these individuals mentioned, "[I]t never worked out that I could be [at the senior center] when [registration] was supposed to be done ... It was a limitation ... so this worked out very well for me." The other individual who acknowledged convenience had participated in the SFMNP prior to the intervention. She described, "I [went] to the senior center, and they give out the vouchers ... I haven't been going there for a while ... because I got ... sick, and I couldn't get to the building." These statements reaffirm that potential barriers to SFMNP access exist for homebound older adults. In-home application assistance addressed awareness and reduced barriers so that low-income homebound seniors could take advantage of benefits for which they were eligible.

Improvements in fruit and vegetable intake

In addition to capturing information about overall fruit and vegetable intake, determining if interviewees actually were able to consume home-delivered offerings was of interest. Indeed, most interviewed clients reported consuming all or most of the home-delivered fresh fruits and vegetables. Three interviewees reported eating half or less of the fresh vegetables they received. Two of these individuals cited food preferences or difficulties in eating certain vegetables. For example, one interviewee stated, "I'm not a big vegetable eater to begin with ... The only times I'll have [them] is with the salad ... The other vegetables I have no need of, and I really don't care for them that much anyway." A third interviewee, who was questioned via proxy, asserted a dislike of fruit and did not consume any of the fresh fruit delivered to him. Nevertheless, this particular client's spouse claimed to eat these items, so no fruit was wasted. This feedback suggested that even if a minority of clients did not eat the fresh fruits and vegetables themselves, other outlets for the home-delivered offerings may have existed.

In spite of efforts on part of the authors and the NBCFM market manager to order easy-to-eat items, some interviewees reported difficulty in preparing or consuming home-delivered fresh fruits and vegetables. Three interviewees mentioned challenges with fresh vegetables, whereas only one client reported challenges with fresh fruit. Such difficulties may have been difficult to avoid since interviewees reported coping with challenges, like poor dentition, differently. Whereas one interviewee noted difficulties in eating harder fruit because of dental issues, another interviewee stated, "I got my teeth out, but I can still eat ... peaches and plums and all that kind of stuff." Although the intervention aimed to be sensitive to clients' needs, this finding underscored the broad range of ability and impairment present in the homebound senior population.

Qualitative assessments of fruit and vegetable intake were important to include in the interviews because of shortcomings of quantitative measures. Nine out of 17 found it challenging to recall the fruits and vegetables they had consumed in the past week. Since data from the BRFSS may have been unreliable, it is not presented. However, most interviewees reported changes in their intake, with 65 percent reporting a change in fruit consumption and 56 percent reporting a change in vegetable intake. Change was defined broadly either as an increase or decrease in intake or as an introduction of new foods into the diet; interviewees most frequently stated that their intake had increased. One client noted, "I'm definitely sure [the intervention] made a big difference because I wasn't used to eating that much fruit. I eat fruit, but not like that ... I really took note of it too, so I definitely have to start buying more fruit." Comments like these suggested how for some clients, even a short-term intervention could spark intentions for future dietary behaviors.

Satisfaction and desire to participate again

While multiple dimensions of intervention satisfaction could have been measured, the interview sought to understand interviewees' perceptions of quality and variety of home-delivered fresh fruits and vegetables. The majority of interviewees rated quality of home-delivered fresh fruits and vegetables as good, very good, or excellent. Most interviewed clients rated variety in a similar fashion as well;

however, positive ratings of fruit variety were slightly higher than those for vegetable variety.

Based on these perceptions and other comments made throughout the interviews, it was apparent that most interviewees had positive impressions of the intervention. When asked explicitly, all interviewees stated they would participate in the intervention if it were offered again. Satisfaction in terms of quality and variety of offerings was not necessarily the only driver of desire to continue participation. Indeed, one client shared, "[The intervention] helped me out food-wise as far as blending things in that helped me extend my food situation … I'll manage, but I'm going to miss [the intervention]."

Limitations

Although tracking and assessment of intervention reach, implementation, and effectiveness provided rich information, there were several limitations to the intervention evaluation.

First, while the study provides data about program effectiveness, some design factors may affect the interpretability of results. For example, the retrospective and un-controlled nature of the study limits interpretations about change in respondents' consumption of fresh fruit and vegetables during the intervention period, which was one of the primary outcomes under study, as does reliance on self-report measures. Second, while interview questions assessed qualitative and quantitative changes in consumption, some responses may be biased. Interviewees' sense of the "correct" answer, known as social desirability bias, may have influenced qualitative responses. Self-reported memory problems may have diminished accuracy of quantitative responses. Although the multi-method approach and triangulation of these data provides a richer and more complete picture, it is still important to acknowledge the potential issues with both the qualitative and quantitative measures used.

Third, while all eligible MOWGNB clients were contacted to complete an interview, recruitment methods may have introduced selection bias. Although enrolling study participants via telephone was most feasible, the convenience sample recruited may have been systematically different from those who were unreachable or declined participation. This is especially notable given that those individuals who may have a harder time speaking on the phone may also have been the ones who would have had more challenges using the fresh fruit and vegetables.

Fourth, while program implementation incorporated lessons from past models, its scale and duration may have limited program impact. Given the relatively small quantity of fresh fruit and vegetables delivered over just seven weeks, it is possible that the intervention's dose was not high enough to elicit meaningful change in fruit and vegetable intake. Although program satisfaction was quite high, it may have been even higher with a higher dose intervention. Still, unanimous support of the intervention from interviewed clients suggests that despite its small scale and short duration, the pilot intervention was well received.

Lessons learned

As more seniors live independently, it is important to understand how community resources may be mobilized to meet the needs of older adults, especially those with functional impairments like the homebound seniors who receive home-delivered meals.

Each component of the intervention reported here relied upon partnerships with administering agencies and community organizations, and the infrastructure is in place to continue the project past the intervention period. Although we were not able to continue in-home SFMNP application assistance given the labor-intensive nature of the process, the fresh fruit and vegetable home delivery has continued. The NBCFM has donated the produce and the other necessary infrastructure is in place. An important take away is that creating interventions that use existing resources and relationships greatly increases the long-term sustainability of the project.

This study identifies a potential coverage gap in SFMNP and adds to the currently small body of literature on this federal nutrition assistance program. In addition, the intervention demonstrates that by providing in-home registration assistance, low-income homebound seniors can gain access to benefits. With permission from local SFMNP-administering agencies, coupons can be redeemed off-site from farmers' markets. This thereby increases convenience and access of the SFMNP for participants with limited mobility.

Looking to the future

The significance of the intervention presented here goes beyond filling a gap in the literature on homebound seniors' access to the SFMNP. The SFMNP itself is a critical federal nutrition assistance program that increases affordability of fresh fruits and vegetables for low-income seniors. However, given its very specific focus and restricted window of operation, the program's potential impact on homebound seniors' nutritional intake is limited. Similar appraisals may be made about the broader intervention described, irrespective of funding source.

Developments in federal nutrition assistance policy that have unfolded since the intervention's completion point to opportunities to have broader impact, particularly for homebound seniors of low income. In July 2015, the USDA announced a proposal to allow homebound seniors participating in the Supplemental Nutrition Assistance Program (SNAP) to use their benefits to pay for home-delivered groceries (USDA Food and Nutrition Service, 2015c). SNAP is the largest federal nutrition assistance program, and unlike the SFMNP, seasonal restrictions and narrow purchasing limitations do not apply (USDA Food and Nutrition Service, 2015b). Under the proposal, certain entities would be authorized to deliver groceries and accept SNAP benefits as payment (USDA Food and Nutrition Service 2015c). Many such entities may already serve the proposal's prospective beneficiaries with home-delivered meals funded through Title IIIC of the OAA. Once finalized, this policy development will likely make use of synergies between two federal programs, keeping in the spirit of the intervention described in this chapter. As a result, low-income homebound seniors may experience improved access to a range of foods that is broader than what can be achieved through linking farm to home.

Acknowledgements

For providing funds for the produce and invaluable assistance with the deliveries, we thank Johnson and Johnson, the Rutgers Cooperative Extension, and the New Brunswick Farmers' Market, particularly Carolina Mueller and William Hallman. We thank Linda Higgins at the Middlesex County Office of Aging and Disabled Services for her flexibility and assistance with Senior Farmers' Market Nutrition Program enrollment. We thank Elijah's Promise for their willingness to store the fresh fruit and vegetables. We thank Shareka Fitz, program director at Meals on Wheels in Greater New Brunswick, for helping to coordinate the deliveries, and the delivery volunteers who delivered the fresh fruits and vegetables directly to the clients. We thank Nicholas Shatan and the Ralph W. Vorhees Center for Civic Engagement for creating the map used in this chapter. Finally, we thank the clients of Meals on Wheels in Greater New Brunswick for participating in the program and sharing their experiences with us.

References

Biemiller, L. 2009. "Notes from academe: Rutgers reaches out to make a mercado." *The Chronicle of Higher Education*, October 18. Available online at http://chronicle.com/article/Rutgers-Reaches-Out-to-Make/48816 (accessed July 31, 2014).

Centers for Disease Control and Prevention. 2012. *Behavioral Risk Factor Surveillance System Questionnaire*. Atlanta, GA. Available online at www.cdc.gov/brfss/questionnaires/pdf-ques/2013-brfss_english.pdf (accessed July 31, 2014).

Cuite, C., and Dixon, S. 2015. *Farmers Markets and CSAs in New Brunswick: A Report of the Working Together for a Food Secure New Brunswick Community Food Assessment*. New Brunswick, NJ.

Cuite, C., Dahwan, M., and Fitz, S. 2013. *Increasing Food Security for the Homebound Elderly in New Brunswick*. Available online at http://humeco.rutgers.edu/documents_pdf/news/snapreport.pdf (accessed July 31, 2014).

Gergerich, E., Shobe, M., and Christy, K. 2015. "Sustaining our nation's seniors through federal food and nutrition programs." *Journal of Nutrition in Gerontology and Geriatrics* 34 (3): 273–291.

Hallman, W., Byrd-Bredbenner, C., Cuite, C., McWilliams, R., Senger-Mersich, A., Sastri, N., and Netterville, L. (in preparation). "Nutritional Adequacy and Quality of the Home Food Supply Quality of Elderly Recipients of Home Delivered Meals."

Institute of Medicine. 2012. *Nutrition and Healthy Aging in the Community: Workshop Summary*. Washington, DC: The National Academies Press.

Johnson, D., Beaudoin, S., Smith, L.T., Beresford, S.A., and LoGerfo, J.P. 2004. "Increasing fruit and vegetable intake in homebound elders: The Seattle Senior Farmers' Market Nutrition Pilot Program." *Preventing Chronic Disease*. Available online at www.cdc.gov/pcd/issues/2004/jan/03_00010a.htm (accessed July 31, 2014).

Kunkel, M., Luccia, B., and Moore, A. 2003. "Evaluation of the South Carolina Senior Farmers' Market Nutrition Education Program." *Journal of the American Dietetic Association* 103 (7): 880–883.

Lawson, L., Drake, L., and Fitzgerald, N. 2016. "Foregrounding community-building in community food security: A case study of the New Brunswick Community Farmers Market and Esperanza Garden." In A. Morales and J. Dawson (eds.), *Cities of Farmers: Problems, Possibilities and Processes of Producing Food in Cities.* Iowa City: University of Iowa Press.

McCormack, L., Nelson Laska, M., Larson, N., and Story, M. 2010. "Review of the nutritional implications of farmers' markets and community gardens: A call for evaluation and research efforts." *Journal of the American Dietetic Association,* 110: 399–408.

Meals on Wheels America. 2015. United States [fact sheet]. Available online at www. mealsonwheelsamerica.org/docs/default-source/fact-sheets/senior-fact-sheet-national. pdf?sfvrsn=2 (accessed October 31, 2015).

Meals on Wheels in Greater New Brunswick n.d. Program information [brochure]. Available online at http://mowgnb.org/pdf/mowgnb_brochure.pdf (accessed July 31, 2014).

Middlesex County n.d. Nutrition services. Available online at www.co.middlesex.nj.us/ Government/Departments/CS/Pages/Aging%20and%20Disabled%20Services/ Nutrition-Services.aspx (accessed July 31, 2014).

Napili, A. and Colello, K. 2015. *Older Americans Act: FY2015 Appropriations Overview.* Available online at www.hsdl.org/?view&did=762245 (accessed October 31, 2015).

New Brunswick Community Food Alliance n.d. *Our History.* Available online at www. nbfoodalliance.org/about/history (accessed July 31, 2014).

Sinnett, S., Bengle, R., Reddy, S., Johnson, M.A., and Lee, J.S. 2009. "The USDA Senior Farmers' Market Nutrition Program: Inclusion of older adults participating in the Home-Delivered Meal Program in northeast Georgia [abstract]." *Journal of Nutrition Education and Behavior* 41(4S): S1.

Smith, L., Johnson, D.B., Beaudoin, S., Monsen, E.R., and LoGerfo, J.P. 2004. "Qualitative assessment of participant utilization and satisfaction with the Seattle Senior Farmers' Market Nutrition Pilot Program." *Preventing Chronic Disease,* 1 (1): 1–11.

State of NJ Department of Health. 2015. *Senior Farmers' Market Nutrition Program.* Available online at www.state.nj.us/health/fhs/wic/farmermktsenior.shtml (accessed October 31, 2015).

U.S. Census Bureau. 2015. *State and County Quick Facts: New Brunswick (city), New Jersey.* Available online at http://quickfacts.census.gov/qfd/states/34/3451210.html (accessed October 31, 2015).

USDA Food and Nutrition Service. 2006. "7 CFR Part 249 Senior Farmers' Market Nutrition Program regulations; Final rule." *Federal Register* 71 (238), 74618–74654.

USDA Food and Nutrition Service. 2007. "7 CFR Part 249 Senior Farmers' Market Nutrition Program Regulations: Announcement of approval and compliance date, with technical amendment." *Federal Register* 72 (56): 13671.

USDA Food and Nutrition Service. 2014. *Senior Farmers' Market Nutrition Program: Overview.* Available online at www.fns.usda.gov/sfmnp/overview (accessed July 31, 2014).

USDA Food and Nutrition Service. 2015a. *Senior Farmers' Market Nutrition Program 2014 Profile.* Available online at www.fns.usda.gov/sites/default/files/sfmnp/

SFMNP%20Profile%20for%20Participating%20State%20Agencies%20-%20FY2014.
pdf (accessed October 31, 2015).

USDA Food and Nutrition Service. 2015b. *Supplemental Nutrition Assistance Program: Eligibility*. Available online at www.fns.usda.gov/snap/eligibility (accessed October 31, 2015).

USDA Food and Nutrition Service. 2015c. "Supplemental Nutrition Assistance Program: Implementation of the Agricultural Act of 2014 purchasing and delivery services for the elderly and disabled." *Federal Register* 80 (135): 41442–41447.

U.S. DHHS Administration for Community Living. n.d. Administration on Aging (AoA): Nutrition Services (OAA Title IIIC). Available online at www.aoa.gov/AoA_Programs/HPW/Nutrition_Services/index.aspx (accessed October 31, 2015).

Van Duyn, M. and Pivonka, E. 2000. "Overview of the health benefits of fruit and vegetable consumption for the dietetics professional: Selected literature." *Journal of the American Dietetic Association* 100: 1511–1521.

Webber, D., Balsam, A., and Oehlke, B. 1995. "The Massachusetts Farmers' Market Coupon Program for low-income elders." *The Art of Health Promotion* [newsletter] 9 (4): 251–253.

Part II

Building local food system sustainability

7   What grows in East New York

'East New York Farms!' and expectations of urban agriculture

Sarita Daftary-Steel, Christine M. Porter,
Suzanne Gervais, David Vigil, and Daryl Marshall

> How beautiful it is, and how honorable it is when someone from Jamaica goes to Pauline or goes to her sister and [buys] callaloo… and you could see the joy in that interaction. And where do you have that? It's so beautiful, that out of East New York you get to have that joy, that possibility…For me, I'm looking forward to teaching people what grows in East New York.
>
> (Kele Nkhereanye, community educator and
> mini-grantee with East New York Farms!)

East New York grows East New York Farms!

East New York is a culturally rich, ethnically diverse and economically disadvantaged community located in eastern Brooklyn. Our 183,971 residents are predominantly Black (52 percent) and Hispanic (37 percent), with approximately 35 percent immigrant households. Our community faces problems that are symptoms of historical discrimination: high levels of violence, high poverty rates (32 percent), high unemployment (14 percent), and one of the highest rates of incarceration in the city. Many residents struggle to find and afford fresh healthy food, and this is reflected in high rates of diabetes, obesity, and heart disease (King et al. 2015).

In the mid-1990s, East New York was slowly recovering from decades of neglect and disinvestment spurred by racially discriminatory housing policies and real estate tactics that exploited these policies. During the 1960s and 1970s, large numbers of white residents left East New York for the suburbs and for new developments on the city's outskirts that were at times in law and in practice only available to whites. East New York became riddled with abandoned properties. As these were knocked down or burned down in the 1970s and 1980s, they became vacant lots that gave birth to dozens of community gardens. By the 1990s some redevelopment efforts had begun in East New York. In particular the Nehemiah Homes project led by East Brooklyn Congregations, which constructed thousands of single-family homes, spurred a substantial repopulation of East New York with homeowners (NYU Furman Center 2015).

The East New York Farms! Project (ENYF) began operations 1998. In 1995, the Pratt Center for Community Development worked with local organizations to initiate a series of community opinion forums. They asked residents to identify both needs and existing resources in East New York. Needs mentioned included more safe public spaces and green spaces, more income generating opportunities, more retail convenience – especially fresh food – and better opportunities for youth. Resources noted included our abundance of community gardens – over 65 – in fact, more than any other neighborhood in New York City. Participants also mentioned the gardeners themselves, residents who had the vision and commitment to turn vacant lots into vibrant gardens, and they mentioned youth, over one-third of the population in our community, and the potential they held.

Through a coalition of organizations and local residents called the East New York Planning Group, the East New York Farms! Project came together as a way to further develop these resources to meet community needs. For more details on ENYF's history and growth, see the project's comprehensive case study online (Daftary-Steel and Gervais 2014). Since 2007, ENYF has operated as a program of United Community Centers (UCC), one of the founding members of the East New York Planning Group and an organization with a more than 60-year history of engaging residents in fostering social change in East New York.

East New York Farms! helps grow East New York

Building on community assets identified through that planning process, ENYF grew steadily to a program that now engages 33 youth interns, over 150 local gardeners, and hundreds of volunteers in growing food and strengthening community through a network of 40 community gardens and more than 20 backyard gardens throughout East New York. ENYF staff supports them and they support ENYF and each other. Today, the goals of ENYF are to:

- Make fresh, healthy food more available and affordable in our community.
- Promote a healthier local and global environment by producing our own food using organic methods and working with other local growers.
- Build our local economy by creating markets for local gardeners and other producers to sell their products.
- Use food as a means to engage community members in taking action and leadership roles as youth interns, gardeners, garden coordinators, garden advocates, community educators, advisory committee and board members, or simply conscious consumers.
- Use food as a means to build community by growing, cooking, and celebrating different food traditions and bringing together people across barriers of age, race, ethnicity, gender, and religion.

ENYF's major program areas include:

> *Gardener support and food production*: ENYF works with a network of backyard gardens and community gardens throughout East New York. We support gardeners with technical aspects of growing and selling food, as well

as building participation in and advocating for their gardens. Staff members provide over 200 hours in individual technical assistance to gardeners in addition to organizing 15 group workshops annually. ENYF also manages three urban farms – the UCC Youth Farm, Fresh Farm, and the Pink Houses Community Farm – where we practice intensive sustainable agriculture methods that can be replicated throughout the community.

Farmers markets and food access: Through two community-run farmers markets ENYF works to make fresh food available and affordable while creating opportunities for entrepreneurs and creating places for neighbors to gather with regular community programming like performances, cooking contests, workshops, and activities for kids (Daftary-Steel 2014). At times in the past we have also operated subscription farm share programs. Through a Steering Committee established as part of our work with the Food Dignity Project, we offer mini-grants to East New York residents who are developing projects to increase food access in the community.

Youth internship program: Each March through November, 33 youth from East New York participate in our intensive internship program. They are involved in all aspects of running a half-acre organic farm and its vendor stand at the farmers market, as well as providing support to other gardens throughout East New York. Many youth stay involved for multiple years as "returning interns" who help lead the program and train new interns (Daftary-Steel 2015).

Community education: Community Educators are residents trained in partnership with a citywide organization, Just Food, to provide cooking demonstrations, presentations, and gardening workshops to educate our neighbors about what's happening around food and health in East New York and how to get involved. Through the UCC Youth Farm, we also provide on-farm education for approximately 1,000 visitors and volunteers of all ages, including many youth from local schools and after-school programs.

Dodging the 'silver bullet' of unrealistic expectations of urban agriculture

In East New York, and across the country, urban agriculture (UA) has emerged as a promising way to address many important issues, including growing food for local communities, preserving open space, promoting health, and developing local leaders. What counts as possible benefits of UA depends in part on what activities count as UA. Here, we use the New York City Five Borough Farm project's definition, as it is grounded in the experience of dozens of New York UA operations:

Urban agriculture can be defined as growing fruits, herbs and vegetables, and raising animals in cities, a process that is accompanied by many other complementary activities such as processing and distributing food, collecting and reusing food waste and rainwater, and educating, organizing and employing local residents

(Cohen et al. 2012: 13).

A worrying expectation, however, has developed for UA to meet these important and ambitious goals while also being financially sustainable without outside funding. We call this expectation the *unattainable trifecta of urban agriculture*—the myth that UA can, without long-term funding investments or major policy shifts, simultaneously do three things that are each hard enough to do on their own:

1   Provide good food to people with limited financial resources at prices they can afford.
2   Provide job training, work experience, and/or leadership development for people typically excluded from employment.
3   Generate income for producers and create jobs funded by profits from sales.

While ENYF's wide-ranging goals and activities hint at the depth and breadth of our project, we understand that UA is not a silver bullet, nor can it achieve its greatest potential in terms of social impacts without outside funding that is often substantial and ongoing. Below we examine some of the challenges that arise as UA organizations work to meet each of these expectations. We discuss this set of expectations more fully in Daftary-Steel, Herrera, and Porter (2015), from which this section draws.

Expectation 1: provide good food to people with limited financial resources at prices they can afford

Like many UA endeavors, ENYF explicitly aims to create access to fresh, *good* food for people who would otherwise struggle to afford it. "Good" food being, per the Wallace Center's definition, "healthy, green, fair and affordable." (National Good Food Network 2015). But achieving this goal is complicated by at least two significant barriers. First, while on average Americans spend a lower proportion of their incomes on food than people in other nations, the U.S. also has one of the highest inequality rates of Global North nations, so what many people in the U.S. can afford to spend on food is very little. Half of households in East New York have incomes of $40,000, with nearly 30 percent earning $20,000 or less, even though the area's official employment rate is 85 percent (NYU Furman Center 2014: 80). A family of four that receives the maximum annual Supplemental Nutrition Assistance Program (SNAP) benefit of $7,788 gets an average of $7.13 *per family meal* (USDA 2015). Other food assistance programs, while helpful, are even smaller in scale. For example, the Farmers' Market Nutrition Program (FMNP), which provides vouchers for seniors and women with children to use at farmers markets, and is used extensively at the East New York Farmers Market, provides only $20 – $24 per year per household. As a result, if our UA operations charged the actual cost of producing our locally grown, organic fresh fruits and vegetables, our food would be unaffordable for most people in our neighborhood.

Second, our largest national food and farm policy programs do not support the production or consumption of fresh, healthy food. The striking dissonance between our federal guidelines about what we should eat versus federal supports for what food we produce is noted with each federal "farm bill" (e.g., Barrington 2011; Physicians Committee for Responsible Medicine 2007). USDA dietary guidelines urge that we fill half of our plates with fruits and vegetables, yet federal spending on agriculture allocates a fraction of a percent to fruit and vegetable production. Producers of these so-called "specialty crops" then need to recoup their full cost of production, unlike those growing heavily subsidized commodity crops such as corn and soy. For example, according to the Environmental Working Group farm subsidy database of USDA-provided data, from 1995 to 2012, corn producers received a total of $84.4 billion in subsidies as compared to $262 million for apple producers (Environmental Working Group 2015). While the good food that ENYF produced obtained some federal support during that time in the form of competitive short-term grants, we got zero dollars in annual federal subsidies.

The combined realities of low incomes and comparatively high produce prices mean that the unhealthy options are too often the most affordable and accessible options for millions of Americans living in communities like East New York.

Expectation 2: provide job training, work experience, and/or leadership development for people typically excluded from employment

As the research of the Five Borough Farm Project (Five Borough Farm 2015) notes, UA has the potential not just to feed people but to contribute to youth development, education, and job readiness. The need for innovative approaches to job training, job creation, income generation, and employment pathways is clear. One in seven young people in the US is "disconnected," not in school and not working (Salemson 2012). In East New York, this rate jumps to 25 percent (Measure of America 2014: 3). Nearly 4 million Americans suffer from long-term unemployment, defined as such because they have been looking for work and have been unemployed for more than 6 months (Kasperkevic 2014). Because UA is often community-based, therapeutic and linked to local organizations, combining UA with job training, leadership development, or employment of the "least employable" (such as the differently abled, people with criminal records, or "disconnected" young people) is a natural fit. However, both experienced staff and adequate staff-to-participant ratios are needed to provide appropriate training that goes beyond acquiring technical skills. In addition to helping participants develop a range of leadership skills, UA job training programs often need to compensate for deficits in math, reading and writing skills due to poor quality public schools, and to address social and emotional needs, on top of teaching technical farming skills that are often completely new to participants.

Each year ENYF provides hundreds of hours of leadership development and job training for 33 youth, ages 13–18, through our nine-month paid internship program (Daftary-Steel 2015). But the challenges many of our youth interns face each day are not just about accessing affordable fruits and vegetables, but about surviving. At any given time, interns in our program may be living in shelters, struggling academically, worried about their safety traveling to and from school and work, suffering physical or verbal abuse at home, navigating the challenges of immigration, dealing with the frustration of being stopped-and-frisked frequently, battling mental health issues, or just coping with the daily challenges and indignities of being poor. A question that funders, researchers, students, and reporters often ask us about our youth program is if our interns now eat more vegetables than they did before the program. The short answer is almost certainly yes, but that isn't the most salient point nor is it primarily how we assess our work. We do, however, judge ourselves by our ability to help youth see themselves as valuable, capable people, well-prepared to make thoughtful choices to improve their own lives and the world around them (Daftary-Steel 2015: 17).

Creating opportunities for the many people chronically excluded from our workforce is a responsibility that our country cannot ignore. But expecting that urban farms could or should do this without long-term investments of outside funds for that purpose is unrealistic, all the more so if we are also expecting people new to farming and even to working in the formal economy to produce enough to sell at a profit.

Expectation 3: generate income for producers and create jobs funded by profits from sales

In our experience, this expectation arises from both UA organizers and proponents themselves as well as from funders. For example, a potential funder that visited ENYF praised our strong leadership by community members, our highly successful youth internship program, and our community market, but was disappointed with the revenue generated from produce sales to our community. Their representative suggested that we should consider selling a portion of our produce to some high-end restaurants to generate more income, or if we did not want to take any of our current land out of community-directed production, perhaps we should start a rooftop farm on the top of our building and direct this produce to restaurants. A rooftop farm focused on high-end products would have involved adding or shifting a significant amount of staff time and required far more capital than we had or than the funder would offer. A rooftop location would also move our work literally away from easy community access and view. Since garden-grown produce sells out at our markets each week, directing any of it to restaurants would interfere with our goal of meeting the need for fresh produce in our community. We gently explained why neither of these revenue-generating strategies was practical for us or a fit with our mission. We were not invited for a full proposal and they suggested that we reach out to them if we were considering expanding our economic development focus in the future.

At ENYF, economic development is among our goals. More than 45 gardeners in our network, two regional farmers, and 15 craft and prepared food vendors join our youth interns in selling at our two farmers markets from June through November. Our large Saturday market and a Wednesday farm stand collectively generated over $110,000 in sales last year, with over $50,000 earned by local residents, and $20,000 in sales of urban-grown produce. Customers redeemed nearly $60,000 worth of food assistance dollars through government programs like FMNP, SNAP, the New York City Healthbucks Program, and New York State FreshConnect Program. Vendors at our market earn supplemental – and in some cases primary – income, but we have no illusion that the internships created through our youth program, much less long-term living wage jobs, could be supported by the sales we currently achieve through our half-acre youth-and-staff run farm, likely the most intensively farmed space in our network of East New York gardens.

Making a farming business profitable, even moderately profitable, is hard. The median farm operator in the US incurs a net loss (Economic Research Service 2014). Notably, urban gardens or small sustainable farms are *not* less efficient or less productive than large farms; the opposite appears to be the case (IAASTD 2009: 151). Research by some of our partners in a national action research project called Food Dignity, where gardeners in Ithaca, New York, and in Laramie, Wyoming, are quantifying their home and community garden harvests, has found that average harvest yields per area in community gardens are on par with yield rates from commercial farms (Conk and Porter 2016).

Though producing and selling food in UA operations does generate some revenue and can be an important source of unrestricted funds for non-profit farms, for those aiming to provide other benefits to their communities, such as affordable food to their neighborhoods and jobs for the least "employable," that revenue will not cover operational costs, much less generate a profit. ENYF for example earns about 2 percent of its operating budget through produce sales. City Slicker Farms, a UA organization operating in West Oakland for nearly 15 years to date, reports covering about 4 percent of its operational costs that way (City Slicker Farms 2013: 3). Like ENYF, City Slicker Farms focuses on selling produce within its community at affordable prices and runs related programs that generate no income, such as helping community and backyard gardeners grow their own food, and providing job training and leadership development for teenagers.

Most UA organization operators know that they cannot meet all three of these expectations simultaneously. But it seems many are reluctant to admit that, at least publicly. Such an admission can look like a failure of their organization or enterprise, rather than realistic statement about the failures of broader systems and what kind of support is required to enable UA operations to address some of these failures (Lawson 2005). Some practitioners are speaking up and trying to craft a better-informed narrative of what makes an UA project successful (Johnson 2014). Urban agriculture, in the words of LaDonna Redmond, requires "becoming organizers and not food science providers" (DeLind 2014: 5).

Lessons from ENYF successes, struggles, and strategies

Despite the unrealistic expectations to which UA projects are often held, ENYF has survived and by many measures thrived as a community-driven effort for almost 20 years. We have learned a great deal about how to sustain this type of work, and offer some lessons from our experience.

Lesson 1: remember who you are and where you come from

ENYF started as the result of a community planning process focused on identifying needs, assets, and opportunities in East New York. ENYF did not start because East New York residents were primarily concerned about demonstrating the potential of urban agriculture and promoting sustainable lifestyles, nor because they were uniquely focused on food as the only important issue in their community. *ENYF started because our community was struggling*, and looking for a way to use the tools we had to build something that could improve quality of life. This has proved a useful lens for maintaining our focus and our *accountability to the East New York community*.

Given the impossibility of reaching the "unattainable trifecta" of UA goals described above without significant and sustainable outside financial support, ENYF made and continues to make choices to focus on two parts of this trifecta: providing good food at prices our neighbors can afford; and providing job training, work experience, and leadership development for our community. We work to make good fresh food available and affordable in our community by growing it in the spaces we manage with our staff and youth interns and supporting neighbors in doing the same in their community and backyard gardens, and creating community markets. We also use food as a means to build leadership in our community, working most intensively with youth in our structured internship program but also substantially with adults who participate in training around sustainable agriculture, marketing, community education, grant-writing, meeting facilitation, and more. We recognize the great need for income generating opportunities in our community, and strive to create them where we reasonably can. Youth are paid stipends, market gardeners earn supplemental income at our farmers market, community educators earn stipends for teaching gardening and cooking workshops, and many gardeners save money on groceries by growing their own food. We also recognize this robust range of programming requires external financial support, in the same way that our public education institutions need external financial support, and we are committed to ongoing fundraising efforts.

We make this choice explicitly. As in the earlier story about a visit from a potential funder, ENYF staff members are asked fairly often if we could sell some of our produce to high-end buyers to subsidize the cost of other produce that we sell to our community at low prices. The realistic answer is, not really. The UCC Youth Farm, our half-acre farm cultivated by youth interns, sells about $10,000 worth of produce each year. If we took a quarter of that produce, quadrupled the price, and sold it to restaurants, we could make an extra $7,500, towards a total annual budget of $430,000. While ENYF programs are so integrated that it's hard to truly separate costs, we estimate that the UCC Youth Farm costs alone are about $38,000 per year. This does not include youth program labor, but does include farm manager labor and time spent leading educational tours and hosting volunteers, since we cannot imagine running our farm and refusing to let a local first grade class visit, for example. Staff salaries are low for New York City ($35 – 45K per year), and overhead is low because we pay no rent for our basement office space. So, for that added $7,500 gained from restaurant sales, we would have to shift our mission, start a new program area focusing staff time on securing and delivering to high-end restaurants that are generally far from our farm, and make our market stand in our own community, which quickly sells out of most items, 25 percent emptier.

We also make this choice because *we understand where our work sits in the history and trajectory of our community*. East New York is among many communities of color still feeling the deep wounds of decades of public and private disinvestment – spanning from the 1930s arguably to the present day, in the forms of redlining, blockbusting, restrictive covenants, planned shrinkage, and predatory lending, among others. This disinvestment formed the updated face of structural racism that limited wealth creation in the North for people whose wealth creation opportunities had already been blocked by enslavement in the South and the Caribbean, followed by Black Codes, land and property loss through domestic terrorism and federal discrimination, and Jim Crow laws. Our ongoing reality of structural racism, that has been documented in everything from property values to quality of education to racial disparities in sentencing and employment discrimination, has led to vast income gaps and even greater wealth gaps that afflict primarily Black and Latino communities like East New York (see Marwell 2007; Bouie 2015).

Today, this means that when people in East New York want to get together to do something, they can and do bring resources like knowledge, pride, diversity, farming experience, available land, and more, but financial resources and disposable wealth or income are often scarce. Funds from government and private grants represent a small amount of the redistribution that probably should happen and reparations that probably are owed to many East New Yorkers. Needing to apply for grants is not ideal, but if we are willing to put in the extra time to find the funders who will let us do things the way we know best, and we can manage to maintain our focus in the face of misguided suggestions that may come from people who have money to give, we can maintain *a project that is community-led even if it is not exclusively community-funded.*

Our commitment to building ownership, leadership, knowledge, and food access *in East New York* makes it fairly easy to see that a rooftop farming and restaurant supply initiative would have been a distraction from our core work. Using this filter also helps us carefully select only the grant opportunities, partnerships, coalitions, events, interviews and conferences that seem likely to serve the true purpose of our work, even as these opportunities have multiplied with growing attention to urban agriculture and health issues. For example, we have sometimes faced a challenge in explaining to funders and potential funders why we do not plan to expand beyond East New York. The first reason is that focusing on East New York is justifiable because in it live over 180,000 people, each of whom matters, and we have certainly not exceeded our capacity to grow our work within East New York. The second reason is that being rooted in our community is one of the keys to our success. We appreciate opportunities to serve as a model for groups who want to carry out similar projects in their own communities, but they need to form their own projects based on the assets and needs that are unique to their community. Then we can also learn with and from them.

This filter helps us also identify what *are* the right opportunities. For example, when Porter (second author of this chapter), reached out to ENYF in 2010 to invite us to be a partner in the Food Dignity action research project she was developing, we were drawn to the focus on seeking answers to questions that we would help shape, on capturing and sharing our stories the way we wanted them to be told, and on providing leadership development support through training funds and through mini-grants that could help our neighbors to realize their own ideas. It also built on our prior experience with a gardener-managed revolving loan fund that we developed through a partnership with Heifer International.

ENYF participates in networks that stretch beyond East New York when our participation seems likely to contribute to larger change that will benefit our community, and when this participation provides leadership development opportunities for our members. Some examples include co-founding the Brownsville East New York Gardeners Initiative to bolster membership in gardens throughout our neighboring communities; engaging staff, gardeners, and youth interns in delivering testimony at city hearings on land tenure for gardens as part of the New York City Community Garden Coalition; and presenting about our collaborative farm-trials of culturally-relevant crops at regional conferences like the Northeast Organic Farming Association. Recently, ENYF has taken the lead in forming a regional network of youth food justice organizations with the goal of sharing resources, developing young leaders, and working towards policy changes affecting our communities.

Making these choices has been primarily about knowing who we are accountable to and what our strengths and capabilities are, rather than about sticking to narrow definitions of what we can and cannot do. In fact developing programs in ways that combine community and organizational assets in sometimes non-traditional ways has been one of our most successful strategies.

For example, we do substantial work with both youth and adults – which is to say that it is neither youth nor adults who are the "real" focus of our programs. It's both, and we are constantly developing new ways for community members of all ages to engage with ENYF and with each other. Our recently developed *Fresh Farm* is a space where members include elder gardeners, youth alumni, and current youth interns. We've seen them exchanging farming techniques, watering each other's garden beds, and sharing stories. We also offer workshops for both youth and adults – conducted together and separately – to talk about working effectively across generations. Young people and adults build relationships that extend beyond the program and have the opportunity to appreciate the assets each other bring to this work. Additionally, the nature of a youth program with a nine-month internship cycle also means that our interns can't quite have ownership over a garden space in the same way that adults can. Engaging adults facilitates community ownership at another level than we could achieve through our youth program alone. Although leadership development with these two groups requires different strategies, structures and skills, we see residents of all ages, and the relationships between them, as assets for strengthening our work and our community.

We also run our own farm (the UCC Youth Farm) *and* provide assistance to other growers. Many UA groups do one or the other, but for ENYF, combining these efforts helps us reach our goals of increasing local production of affordable fresh food while also demonstrating intensive sustainable production techniques that other growers may want to adopt. This also enables youth interns to have a growing space that they manage, and opportunities to learn from other growers in the neighborhood.

Being steadfast about who we are has meant passing up possible funding opportunities that were an almost-fit, but it ultimately ensured that we stayed true to our mission, which kept staff and members engaged, sustained community support, and eventually helped us build a strong reputation with funders.

Lesson 2: learn intentionally and grow slowly

East New York has seen lofty redevelopment plans amount to nothing; has seen initiatives of non-profit organizations start and end abruptly; and has seen much promised but often little delivered. With our knowledge of this history, we have aimed to build something lasting. This has meant prioritizing continuous learning, and using that learning to inform incremental growth. This has also meant taking fewer risks – or perhaps more calculated ones – and fewer big leaps to start major initiatives that might have to be discontinued when funding runs out, or if we discover these initiatives are not a good fit. Because this ability to demonstrate consistency and stability is incredibly important in East New York, it has been a cornerstone of our success.

Before any plans for ENYF were developed, community organizations partnered with the Pratt Center to hear residents define what they saw as assets and needs in East New York. This process was foundational for ENYF, and we recognize that our community is dynamic and changing. This requires us to *constantly use feedback, suggestions, experiences, and observations* to improve and adjust how we work. We have found that frequent and adaptable ways of evaluating success have served us better than larger, less frequent, and more formal assessments. The changes to programs that resulted from our ongoing learning were often not grand changes – like creating a quarterly calendar to help members plan ahead for workshops and meeting, or having returning interns come to work 15 minutes earlier so that they would be better prepared to lead – but we found that running our core programs basically the same way with *constant small but significant improvements* enabled us to best serve East New York, and take direction from our members and community. This sometimes made fundraising more difficult, as new initiatives are often more attractive to funders than plans to strengthen existing programs or continue effective ones.

Ways that we take direction from our members and community vary by necessity. Structured methods can be important, but we have also found an inverse relation between the structure and depth of participation and the number of people that can make the time to be involved. We learned that we needed to *create multiple ways for members and community to engage in evaluating success and shaping future plans.* In some cases using more flexible models of participation rather than obligatory direct consensus-based decision-making enabled more people to weigh in on the elements of ENYF that matter most to them. For example, for years we held our year-end review and planning meetings as group discussions, but this required people to commit substantial time on a weekend or late evening, and we were concerned, especially as ENYF grew, that a fairly small proportion of members were engaging in the process. So we shifted to an "open house" format, with staff members facilitating different review "stations" by program area over the course of a few hours. Members are free to arrive and leave any time within those few hours, and move through stations as their time and interest allow. It also facilitates more connections among members, since it's now easier them to engage in one-on-one conversations that would be hard to make space for in a focused group discussion. We saw many more members engage in the review process this way.

Being a learning organization also required *being willing to realize that our initial plans were unrealistic.* For example, the first iteration of our youth program in which interns worked directly with gardeners, rather than as part of a coordinated program, did not provide a strong enough group experience to keep youth engaged and motivated, and required too much coordination from gardeners. In order to create a better structure for long-term youth leadership development and support more positive peer relationships, we shifted to a structure in which youth interns work in gardens together in crews of nine, with staff members who coordinate this work and create curriculum to complement it.

Listening, asking questions, and responding in practical ways to feedback from residents have also led us, at times, to adopt strategies even when we have not seen them in practice elsewhere. For example, most farmers markets do not buy, store, and rent equipment for vendors, but we saw early on that doing so would vastly expand opportunities for local entrepreneurs who lacked transportation or funds to purchase their own equipment. We also provide free assistance and supplies for backyard gardeners as well as community gardeners; as far as we know, we are the only organization in New York City that does so. We do it because it creates yet another way for more residents to participate in growing food and community in East New York.

Growing slowly is an important part of our learning approach, so that our programs do not outpace our capacity to learn with and from members and to adapt in response to our learning. It's a practice that can be hard to stick to. For example, after the East New York Farmers Market had been running only a couple of seasons and was still quite small, we submitted a proposal to develop a full-time permanent market site, which we thankfully did not get. We see now that the rent that we would have needed to charge vendors to sustain the site would likely have excluded the gardeners and micro-entrepreneurs who have formed the backbone of our market, and few of them have enough supply and time to run a full-time market stand. As our Saturday market grew, however, we did add a Wednesday market stand in response to customer and vendor feedback. We sometimes pilot limited versions of new programs before having any funding for them, so that we can spend a year or so figuring out if an initiative would work and how, instead of raising money that might "lock" us into activities that may not be as needed or wanted by our community as we thought. Before we started our formal Community Educator training program, we piloted such a program, without dedicated funding, to see how much interest there was and figure out the kinks before seeking funding for the full program that operates today.

Lesson 3: cultivate gardens and relationships

The tangible impacts of our work – the food we are able to grow, the supplemental income gardeners are able to earn, the acres of green spaces that might not exist were it not for gardens – all matter hugely in a community where material needs are substantial. Relationships, and the way in which we sustain these relationships and nurture leadership, are equally important.

Because people are so central to our work, we are always working to *create more ways for people to participate in ENYF*. For example, although we try to encourage as much production as possible on the land available to us in order to meet the great need for fresh food in East New York, we also strive to meet people "where they're at," recognizing that the energy and capacity that people have for food production varies greatly. Our Share Table provides an opportunity for growers of any scale to participate in our markets. Gardeners can drop off produce at the Share Table to be sold by youth interns, and then share proceeds with the youth program. It developed as we learned that only a few gardeners had the time or harvest supply to participate in the market by operating their own stands, but many could contribute to a cooperative table run by youth interns. The Share Table expands income generation opportunities as well as volume and variety of produce at our markets, since the dozens of gardeners who participate in the Share Table hail from a diversity of places including Bangladesh, Guyana, Nigeria, South Carolina and more, and often grow foods they cultivated in those places. Gardeners who participate in the Share Table also build relationships with youth interns and other gardeners and vendors, and tell their neighbors about ENYF.

In addition to building broad engagement, we acknowledge the importance of long-term deep engagement from our core of most committed members. For example, markets often face a challenge of hitting the right balance of adequate supply and demand on each market day. Customers won't come if there aren't enough vendors or products, and vendors often won't come, or won't stay, if there aren't enough customers. Local gardener Johanna Willins and John Ameroso of Cornell Cooperative Extension committed to selling their produce week after week in the first years of building the market to create the consistent supply that was needed to eventually attract customers. Other early joiners like gardeners Eliza Butler, Leila Jamison, Adell Oliver, Gemma Garcia, and Alma Pearson (all members of the East New York Gardeners Association that was active at the time) sold their produce and contributed to variety and supply at the market when it was still quite small. Other dedicated gardener-vendors like Pauline Reid and Dennis and Marlene Wilks have contributed substantial quantities of produce to our markets on a weekly basis for years. Many of our core members have been involved in ENYF for more than 15 years. We try to recognize their contributions and encourage their continued engagement in various ways, like discounts on market fees for vendors who sell consistently, do outreach for the market and attend monthly ENYF meetings, as well as opportunities to further their leadership by attending conferences, trainings, and events that connect them with the food justice movement beyond East New York.

Lesson 4: invest in staff

Hiring and retaining experienced and committed staff members, primarily in roles designed to be full-time and long-term, enables everything else we do at ENYF. Our staff, though a relatively small team of five full-time and two-part time employees, enables our members and volunteers to contribute their vision, commitment, and skills while they also work, raise families, go to school, and meet the many other demands of their lives, including the additional demands poverty creates. Without the ability to pay for quicker or more convenient options, many East New Yorkers spend significant amounts of time doing things that wealthier people are able to avoid, like going to the laundromat, enduring long waits in doctor's offices, enrolling in support programs, or using public transportation exclusively. The time staff can commit is an important resource to facilitate the engagement of others. For example, while committed volunteers worked on developing the UCC Youth Farm for years, it took staff specifically assigned to this project to be able to convert it into a productive farm that could then host dozens of young people in an internship program and more than a thousand visitors and volunteers annually.

Retaining staff helps us to continuously learn from and build on past experiences, and is crucial for building the relationships that anchor our work. Because a deep understanding of "where we come from" is so important, we also prioritize hiring staff with a connection to East New York, especially residents. To do this effectively, we have to make sure our staff recruitment practices are aligned with this goal. We share job opportunities with our local networks first, and have removed educational requirements from our job postings, recognizing that many of our neighbors have not had access to higher education opportunities, and that emphasizing specific skills and relevant experience would better serve our goals.

Box 7.1 Being part of ENYF

Daryl Marshall has been a Community Organizer and Youth Worker with ENYF since 2011, and was involved as a vendor and community educator prior to that. He contributed this reflection about his experience working with community gardeners over the past five years.

Listening, recognizing and trusting are key components to our work with gardeners. Keeping these things in mind as you interact with people is paramount. Growing food is important, but it goes hand in hand with building and maintaining relationships If you want to be welcomed into these open spaces you have to acknowledge and respect gardeners' habits, rituals and culture. Remember as far as they know you can be observing them for a project and never coming back.

Why should one bear all, and give you unlimited access to their space and time? Granted a community garden is not their space technically, it's public property. Unfortunately in a community with limited access to ownership and power, these spaces take on a whole other meaning. This is what it sometimes is about, not just vegetables and extra money, but being able to trust us as an organization that will have their best interest in mind. So when we do introduce them to a researcher, student, volunteer or potential new member, they are more comfortable.

The allure of this work for me was not compensation, but being able to do something meaningful in my community. I could have and wanted to be a fireman, however ageism, tests, and nepotism are some things I might have needed to overcome to become one. However there was no test, and my age or background didn't matter when it was time for me to be hired at ENYF. What did matter was my proven record of already volunteering in my community and my willingness to learn.

Though ENYF has not been able to offer some of the more conventional incentives for staff retention – like high salaries, significant raises, or frequent promotions – we have been able to retain good staff through investments in our team's personal growth and autonomy by making both collaborative and decentralized decisions about our work.

Conclusion

As one of the first-founded and longest-running community urban agriculture projects in the US, ENYF owes its success to the values and consistency that we have maintained as our work has grown and evolved. With our commitment to staying rooted in East New York, we have looked at ways to expand and deepen our future work within the community by focusing on three areas: 1) public housing developments – there is a high need for food access and community-building work, and a dense population of residents to contribute to these efforts; 2) schools – we offer tours and volunteer opportunities to many schools within East New York, as well as developing culinary education programs led by young people; 3) newer immigrant groups – expanding communities of immigrants from West Africa and South Asia bring with them unique food cultures and assets, and we hope to use our gardens and markets to help integrate them into the community. At the same time, we will continue our core programs because we have seen how they offer multiple points of entry and multiple benefits to East New York residents.

Our experience has shown us that *urban agriculture is incredibly valuable even when it is not profitable.* There were many opportunities and incentives along the way to focus too much on the wrong things – to look narrowly at how much food we could produce, how much income we could earn, how quickly we could expand, or to emphasize only quantity but not quality of community involvement. In doing so, we could have squandered some of our deepest and most lasting potential. Urban agriculture as ENYF has practiced it has always been a way to further develop the potential of our community by investing in local leaders and working with them to create something we can all take pride in because we built it together.

We urge philanthropists and policy makers to continue and expand financial support for urban agriculture, so that community-based projects like ours can continue to create physical, social, environmental, and educational benefits as well as food and income, and to work with UA practitioners and others to examine and address root causes of the social issues that have driven farms and gardens to sprout in vacant lots all over the country.

> I hope that everybody that comes to East New York sees where we came from, and where we are today. We're really doing a wonderful job.
>
> (Eliza Butler, coordinator of New Visions Garden
> and East New York Farms! Member)

Acknowledgements

The authors have collaborated since 2011 as part of the five-year action-research collaboration called Food Dignity in which Porter is the Principal Investor and the other authors are co-investigators. Food Dignity is supported by an Agriculture and Food Research Initiative Competitive Grant (no. 2011-68004-30074) from the USDA National Institute of Food and Agriculture (www.fooddignity.org). The views expressed here are the authors' alone.

References

Armstrong, D. 2000. "A survey of community gardens in upstate New York: Implications for health promotion and community development." Health and Place 6 (4): 319–327. Available online at http://nccommunitygarden.ncsu.edu/researchArmstrongSurveyNY HealthCommunityDevelopment.pdf (accessed May 25, 2016).

Barrington, V. 2011. "Wake up to the (secret) Farm Bill." Ecosalon. Available online at http://ecosalon.com/the-secret-farm-bill-food-policy-402/ (accessed December 4, 2015).

Bouie, J. 2015. "How We Built the Ghettos." The Daily Beast. Available online at http://www.thedailybeast.com/articles/2014/03/13/how-we-built-the-ghettos.html (accessed December 3, 2015).

City Slicker Farms. 2013. City Slicker Farms 2013 Annual Report. West Oakland: City Slicker Farms. Available online at http://www.cityslickerfarms.org/sites/default/files/cityslickerfarms_2013_annual_rpt_final_compressed.pdf (accessed May 25, 2016).

Cohen, N., Reynolds, K., and Sanghvi, R. 2012. Five Borough Farm: Seeding the Future of Urban Agriculture in New York City. New York: Design Trust for Public Space in partnership with Added Value.

Conk, S. and Porter, C.M. 2016. "Food gardeners' productivity in Laramie, Wyoming: More than a hobby." American Journal of Public Health 106 (5): 854–856.

DeLind, L. 2014. "Where have all the houses (among other things) gone? Some critical reflections on urban agriculture." Renewable Agriculture and Food Systems 3: 3–7. Available online at http://dx.doi.org/10.1017/S1742170513000525 (accessed May 25, 2016).

Daftary-Steel, S. 2014. Building a Great Farmers Market. Food Dignity Practice Brief 2. Available online at http://fooddignity.org/wp/wp-content/uploads/2014/12/Practical guide-Communitybasedfarmersmarkets-v5_reduced-size.pdf (accessed May 25, 2016).

Daftary-Steel, S. 2015. "Growing Young Leaders in East New York: Lessons from the East New York Farms! Youth Internship Program." Brooklyn, NY: East New York Farms! Available online at http://fooddignity.org/wp/wp-content/uploads/2015/04/ENYF-15-04-28-report-Growing-Young-Leaders.pdf (accessed August 22, 2015).

Daftary-Steel, S. and Gervais, S. 2014. East New York Farms! Retrospective Case Study. Food Dignity project. Available online at http://goo.gl/VVJzlL (accessed September 7, 2016).

Daftary-Steel, S., Herrera, H., and Porter, C. (2015). "The unattainable trifecta of urban agriculture." Journal of Agriculture, Food Systems, and Community Development 6 (1): 19–32. Available online at http://dx.doi.org/10.5304/jafscd.2015.061.014 (accessed May 25, 2016).

Economic Research Service. 2014. Farm Household Income (Historical). United States Department of Agriculture. Available online at http://www.ers.usda.gov/topics/farm-economy/farm-household-well-being/farm-household-income-%28historical%29.aspx#.VD2hjxZhG5I (accessed November 23, 2015).

Environmental Working Group. 2015. EWG Farm Subsidies Database. Available online at http://farm.ewg.org/region.php?fips=00000andprogcode=total (accessed August 22, 2015).

ENYF. 2013. *East New York Farms! Youth Internship Alumni Evaluation Report*. Available online at Available online at www.nrs.fs.fed.us/nyc/local-esources/downloads/2013_ENYF_AlumniReport.pdf (access May 25, 2016).

Five Borough Farm. 2015. Available online at http://www.fiveboroughfarm.org/impact/ (accessed November 23, 2015).

IAASTD. 2009. *Agriculture at a Crossroads*. Johannesburg, South Africa: International Assessment of Agricultural Knowledge, Science and Technology for Development. Global Report. Beverly D. McIntyre, Hans R. Herren, Judi Wakhungu and Robert T. Watson (Eds.)

Johnson, N. 2014. *Urban Farms Won't Feed Us but They Just Might Teach Us*. Available online at http://grist.org/food/urban-farms-wont-feed-us-but-they-just-might-teach-us/ (accessed December 4, 2015).

Kasperkevic, J. 2014. "The ghosts of America's long-term unemployed." *The Guardian*, March 27. Available online at http://www.theguardian.com/money/us-money-blog/2014/mar/27/us-long-term-unemployed-ghosts-economy-jobs (accessed August 22, 2015).

King, L. Hinterland, K., Dragan, K.L., Driver, C.R., Harris, T.G., Gwynn, R.C., Linos, N., Barbot, O., and Bassett, M.T. 2015. *Community Health Profiles 2015*. Brooklyn Community District 5: East New York and Starrett City. Available online at www1.nyc.gov/assets/doh/downloads/pdf/data/2015chp-bk5.pdf (accessed September 7, 2016).

Lawson, L. 2005. *City Bountiful: A Century of Community Gardening in America*. Berkeley: University of California Press.

National Good Food Network. n.d. *Overview and Background*. Wallace Center. Available online at www.wallacecenter.org/ngfn/ (accessed August 22, 2015).

NYU Furman Center. 2014. State of New York City's Housing and Neighborhoods in 2013. New York: NYU Furman Center. Available online at http://furmancenter.org/files/sotc/SOC2013_HighRes.pdf (accessed May 25, 2016).

NYU Furman Center. 2015. Available online at http://furmancenter.org/institute/directory/entry/nehemiah-programeast-brooklyn-congregations-programsouth-bronx-churches-pro (accessed November 23, 2015).

Olson E., Van Wye, G., Kerker, B., Thorpe, L., and Frieden, T.R. 2006. *Take Care East New York and New Lots*. NYC Community Health Profiles, Second Edition. Available online at www1.nyc.gov/assets/doh/downloads/pdf/data/2006chp-204.pdf (accessed September 7, 2016).

Physicians Committee for Responsible Medicine. 2007. *Health v. Pork: Congress Debates the Farm Bill*. Available online at www.pcrm.org/good-medicine/2007/autumn/health-vs-pork-congress-debates-the-farm-bill (accessed May 21, 2015) but is no longer available. Excerpt and graphic now available at http://orangecrateart.tumblr.com/post/461760663 (accessed August 22, 2015).

Salemson, D. 2012. "5.8 million disconnected youth nationally; 350k in NYC." Jobs First NYC. Available online at http://blog.jobsfirstnyc.org/2012/11/58-million-disconnected-youth.html (accessed August 22, 2015).

Social Science Research Council. n.d. *Measure of America*. Available online at http://ssrc-static.s3.amazonaws.com/moa/One_in_Seven_NYC-FINAL2.pdf (accessed November 24, 2015).

USDA. 2015. *Supplemental Nutrition Assistance Program (SNAP): How Much Could I Receive?* Available online at www.fns.usda.gov/snap/how-much-could-i-receive (accessed November 24, 2015).

8 Feeding community

A case study of a shared-use commercial kitchen in eastern Connecticut

Hedley Freake and Phoebe Godfrey

This chapter offers the example of CLiCK, Inc. (Commercially Licensed Co-operative Kitchen), a 501(c)(3) non-profit located in Willimantic, Connecticut and based on co-operative values and committed to a just, locally based, sustainable, and healthy food system, as a model for other communities to address their own social, economic and environmental needs even as we are figuring out how and in what directions CLiCK will continue to grow. CLiCK is not a fixed project; rather, it continues to evolve as we navigate our local assets and deficits in an ongoing attempt to better meet our community's needs. We also use this opportunity to weave together a number of theoretical concepts that act to frame CLiCK's innovative and emerging structure while helping to guide its future development. By way of introduction, these two theoretical concepts are Julian Agyeman's "just sustainability" (2003 and 2013) and Elinor Ostrom's revisioning of the commons (1990 and 1999) that together helped to anchor our practices into a larger social ethos.

A word of disclosure: we are both CLiCK Board members and are therefore biased towards its success. But we seek to be honest as we examine its strengths and weaknesses to ensure that as CLiCK evolves it remains "open" to constructive community critique and input, thereby achieving maximum efficacy. In addition, we are both professors at the nearby University of Connecticut and have involved a number of students with CLiCK. Phoebe Godfrey is a sociologist and Hedley Freake is a nutritional scientist, so we will speak from our distinctive fields and explore the ways in which they have shaped CLiCK while linking back to the framing theoretical concepts that embody its commitment to social / food justice, hence resiliency on a small community level.

To proceed we first describe CLiCK's mission, goals and origins, give a timeline of CLiCK's development and associated grants, and provide a sketch of our current situation. Phoebe will then place CLiCK in a theoretical context, and Hedley will discuss how this context has been applied to CLiCK's emphasis on community health and nutrition. We then explore some of the challenges and successes CLICK has experienced in relation to our two perspectives and in the end integrate our themes to propose how what we have learned and created can be applied elsewhere, while also looking at future steps that CLiCK can take to further achieve its mission.

Mission and goals

> **Grow, Cook, Share**: To grow the vitality of our local economy and community by offering shared use commercial kitchens to farmers and culinary entrepreneurs seeking to create food-based businesses; and to improve the health of our local community by teaching gardening, culinary arts, nutrition and other food-related classes.
>
> (CLiCK n.d.)

CLiCK's two-pronged mission – local food business incubation and nutrition education / culinary training – speaks to the different academic perspectives to be presented in this chapter. CLiCK's mission resulted from a grant received in 2009 that was focused on solutions to local poverty. We spent a year doing community engagement and found that there were two areas of economic need in our region; small rural farmers struggling to sustain their operations and urban un/underemployed individuals seeking ways to develop a meaningful livelihood. There were also a host of associated health issues, mainly within the urban area.

Willimantic, Connecticut (CLiCK is located in Windham which is the surrounding town and county), like many small New England communities, was once a thriving textile mill town. Since the mills closed in the 1980s, it has struggled to find a viable replacement to sustain the local economy. As a result, Willimantic has a poverty rate of over three times the state average. It also has a diverse population, with 40 percent identifying as Hispanic or Latino and the rest a mix of various ethnicities generally classified as "white." Willimantic is surrounded by small farms, some organic, which struggle to compete given the structural inequalities of the industrial food system. These economic concerns are coupled with food security and health issues that result from urban poverty. The town of Windham has 21 percent of its children characterized as food insecure, and the highest rates of childhood obesity in northeastern Connecticut.

Therefore, the idea behind CLiCK was to address these economic and health deficits among both urban and rural populations by creating a shared-use commercial kitchen, as well as a teaching kitchen and community center, committed to social and ecological sustainability. As a shared-use commercial kitchen / food processing center and teaching kitchen, CLiCK's goals are to enable farmers to add value to their products and extend their markets, entrepreneurs to incubate small-scale food businesses, using as many locally sourced products as possible, and community members to benefit from healthy cooking and nutrition education classes. In addition, since CLiCK is a non-profit based on the co-operative values of self-help, self-responsibility, democracy, equality, equity and solidarity, an overarching principle is to pursue these goals in ways that promote social justice on a community level.

Time line

2009 Board Members from the Willimantic Food Co-op recognize the need for small local farmers to have a place to add value to products. A working group is formed.

2010 Poverty reduction grant awarded. Group proposes shared-use kitchen. Year of research confirms need and finds ways to address issues of urban underemployment and poor health.

2011 CLiCK incorporated as a 501(c)(3) non-profit based on co-operative values.

2011–2013 Board meets regularly, does more research to affirm and better define need, applies for grants and searches for a kitchen location.

2014 Funds for a building loaned and a Connecticut Department of Community and Economic Development (DCED) grant for $100,000 and loan for $25,000 awarded (using funds for building as match). A $25,000 USDA Rural Business Enterprise grant received. Purchase of equipment and renovations begin. USDA Local Food Promotion grant for $98,000 awarded plus $21,000 private foundation award to fund teaching kitchen. General Manager hired.

2015 Commercial kitchen opens. Recruitment of members begins. CT Department of Agriculture grant for $43,000 awarded. Construction of teaching kitchen completed. Grounds developed to include community vegetable gardens, orchard, beehives and labyrinth. By November, 14 new businesses have commenced operations; 100 people have attended classes (including summer series for at-risk youth); local organizations including two universities become institutional members; community members become Friends of CLiCK; grant writing and fund-raising efforts ongoing.

2016 CLiCK continues to grow with more new businesses, some old and some new, including one whose co-owner has become the new General Manager. CLiCK has also been able to hire a Community Nutrition Educator using new grant monies from a local foundation and a Processing Outreach and Product Developer funded by the CT Department of Agriculture. These two new positions will help CLiCK to diversify in the directions of community health and nutrition, and processing and product development using locally produced food.

This timeline gives an idea of how long it has taken and how each step and new grant was able to move us along. Although we have been successful with grants, building an income base from the renting of the kitchens has been harder to develop than we originally imagined. As a result one current struggle is cash flow, as all of our grant funds are locked into specific uses. The original plan was that cash flow would come from the use of the commercial kitchen, but this has been slower to develop than anticipated, as we discuss below. The long-term goal for CLiCK is to be self-sustaining with kitchen fees supporting the social service programs, but as we are learning this will take years to build. Having opened in February 2015, we have at the time of this writing (June 2016) been open a year and 4 months and have one central employee, our General Manger, who is responsible for the outreach, programming, user recruitment, daily maintenance, overseeing of the two other part-time employees, as well as all the other aspects of the operation.

Phoebe Godfrey: a sociological perspective

CLiCK's commitment to social / food justice, hence resiliency on a community level, has shaped the ways in which we have approached micro-economic development and nutrition education for a diverse demographic, bringing awareness to the intersecting social conditions of race / ethnicity, class and gender, as well as other social signifiers (religion, legal status, English language proficiency, over commitment, etc.).

This is uncommon for most shared-use kitchens in the New England region, for example Vermont Food Venture Center (Hardwick, VT), Mad River Food Hub (Waitsfield, VT), and Franklin County Community Development Corporation Food Processing Center in Greenfield, Massachusetts. Commonwealth Kitchen, a 501(c)(3) in Boston, does have an emphasis on social justice in terms of doing outreach to those entrepreneurs for whom structural inequality limits their options, but it doesn't offer nutrition education. CLiCK is thus distinguished as being not just a part of the "alternative food" movements but also as being part of the social justice / food sovereignty / community health movements. As Clare Hinrichs states in her introduction to *Remaking the North American Food System* (2007), "Many alternative food initiatives center more on local consumer education and farmer entrepreneurship than social justice issues or needed and challenging policy reforms" (p. 5). CLiCK sees these as inseparable.

CLiCK's commitment emerged not just from the identified needs of our community but also from my exposure to Julian Agyeman's concept of "just sustainabilities" (2003), which has helped me to see that for a community solution to issues of rural and urban poverty and ill health, inequality and justice must be addressed from the start, and not seen merely as add-on goals. Additionally, I have been influenced by Elinor Ostrom's revisioning of Garrett Hardin's concept of the "tragedy of the commons" (1968), even though for both Hardin and Olstom the commons generally involved natural resources. From Hardin's perspective, natural resources held in common invariably end up being over-used and exploited as users compete with each other to maximize their personal returns. His solution was to privatize the commons and manage them though a monetary exchange. In contrast, for Ostrom this "tragedy" was but one possible scenario; she found examples of communities whose use of the their commons do not rely on private or state management but rather are managed, "… from the bottom up to ensure a sustainable, shared management of resources, as well as one that is efficient from an economical point of view" (Felice and Vatiero 2012). Ostrom's examples were again mainly in relation to natural resources, although they did include irrigation systems, demonstrating that the line between what is seen as "natural" resources and what is seen as "social / economic" resources is not clear. For example, Felice and Vatiero make reference to "the Wikipedia community" as demonstrating "a form of successful collective institution of a communal resource (knowledge)" (2012). Likewise, the premise of CLiCK is that the resources, and therefore the costs, of a commercial kitchen are held in common for the benefit of the collective, thereby putting, albeit on a small scale, Agyeman's concept of "just sustainabilities" into practice.

Agyeman (2013: 7) defines "just sustainabilities" as:

- improving our quality of life and well-being;
- meeting needs of both present and future generations (intragenerational and intergenerational equity);
- justice and equity in terms of recognition, process, procedure, and outcomes;
- living within ecosystem limits (also called one planet living).

These goals are reminiscent of the seven co-operative values but speak more directly to the issues of sustainability and fit well with Ostrom's research on the commons (1990). What she found in cases where communities did not turn their commons into a "tragedy" was that they used laws in ways that were beneficial to all, that allowed for the resolution of conflicts and could be collectively changed to meet evolving needs (Felice and Vatiero 2012). Ostrom's recognition of the need to manage a diversity of perspectives and for users of the commons to devise a co-operative strategy (Ostrom 1990: 15) links well with the fact that Agyeman "acknowledges the relative, culturally and place-bound nature of the concept" (2013: 5). Agyeman's emphasis on the plurality of "just sustainabilities" is also supported by Hinrich (2007: 11) who states that "place-based differences need more careful highlighting." Therefore, part of our argument that CLiCK, as a form of the commons, can act as a model for other communities is the recognition that such a model includes place-based awareness focused on "just sustainabilities." In short, it is not possible to separate CLiCK from the place-based needs it has been developed to address. Although poverty exists throughout the country it is important to emphasize that all places have unique characteristics and that the emphasis on "local food" should also include an emphasis on "local social and economic dynamics" in terms of who and what make up a given community and what aspects are held in common.

CLiCK has embodied place-based solutions to our local food needs by carefully identifying those needs and their underlying causes, both on the local and the national levels. As mentioned, CLiCK emerged from the Willimantic Food Co-op Board, Connecticut's oldest member-owned co-op, where small-scale local farmers sell their raw produce. However, for many the return prices barely cover their high costs (Moyer 2015), which is typical for small-scale farmers across the nation and has to do with a combination of the high costs for small-scale organic farm production that often engages in "just" farm and labor practices (treatment of soil / workers / environment … etc.). In contrast, large-scale non-organic industrial farms can bring down prices of competing goods through mass production, extensive use of chemical fertilizers and pesticides, unjust labor and environmental practices and high levels of processing. Food waste is an issue for both types of farming (according to the EPA 20 percent of municipal landfills is food waste) as most raw produce has a short shelf life if it not processed. In fact the original impetus for CLiCK came from the Willimantic Food Co-op's recognition of local food waste and the difficulty of small local organic farms to compete with larger farms because of the lack of value-added options.

These issues were seen to be impediments to local farmer prosperity and so the idea for a shared-use kitchen / processing center was born. However, our surveys indicated that many of these farmers did not want to do the processing / cooking themselves, so the next idea arose for a place that could incubate small businesses, which would purchase from local farmers and develop new food products. In addition, it was proposed that some of these new businesses could help to job train under-skilled and under-employed members of the community, thereby addressing another local economic need. *Then* it was also realized that if some of these new businesses would buy from local farmers and focus on producing healthy food we could indirectly address the local health issues associated with poor nutrition.

Once we had this vision of connecting all the more pressing local (and national) needs, we set about to find a suitable site to create CLiCK. Eventually, we found a building that had space enough for the commercial kitchens and for the construction of a teaching kitchen so we could directly address the local nutrition-associated health issues by offering hands-on cooking and nutrition classes – something not available anywhere in our community. While nutrition classes are offered by the federal Women, Infants, and Children program (WIC) and by Cooking Matters through the national non-profit Share Our Strength, neither is hands-on in a kitchen. Fortunately we also found a member of the community willing to make a loan for the mortgage that also acted as a match for a $100,000 grant from the state for economic development. These ideas and conditions that have gone into creating CLiCK all came from our specific, place-based needs.

Other ways that CLiCK seeks to put the concept of "just sustainabilities" into practice through managing "the commons", as in the kitchen, include creating new possibilities for producing food containing at least 50 percent local ingredients, even for those of modest means. The Connecticut Department of Agriculture reports that less than 2 percent of the food eaten in Connecticut is grown there, so 98 cents of every dollar spent on food leaves the state. The state seeks to increase this to 5 percent, which will require increased local production as well as processing to lengthen the shelf life of locally grown products. The emphasis on local food systems has been central to the sustainability movement, in that they are seen as

> the antithesis to the destructive tendencies of global capitalist industrial agriculture, by offering ecologically sound agriculture practices, support for

small-scale family farms and local economic development, fresher and healthier foods for the consumer, greater democracy and transparency in the food system decision-making, and a more holistic connection between consumer, the farmer, and the rural landscape.

(Agyeman 2013: 60).

This is generally true, however, as Agyeman notes, what is missing is the recognition that "local" can often include segregated spaces in terms of race and social class and therefore an absence of emphasis on social justice and "just sustainabilities." CLiCK's emphasis on creating a non-profit site for processing local foods that are affordable brings together the commitments to "environmental sustainability" and "social justice," thereby ensuring that we are not content to focus on "local" at the expense of "just." In this manner, making a product using organic fair trade ingredients that have been imported might be better than buying "locally" from a farm, large or small, that engages in "unjust" farm and labor practices. As Ageyman (2013: 63) states, "The framing of the local food movement in popular discourse has often confused the ends, which are a more sustainable and socially just food system, with the means: the localization of food production and consumption." While it is not CLiCK's role to prohibit anyone who wishes to use its space to incubate a business from using whatever ingredients they choose, time and effort to be devoted to helping producers make informed decisions that are in line with CLiCK's co-operative and social justice values. In this manner a loose connection can be made to Ostrom's eight principles, which map out how communities can successfully collectively govern and meet their economic needs from their commons just as CLiCK seeks to enable us to do the same (see for example Cox, Arnold, and Tomas, 2010). In addition, since CLiCK received a USDA Local Food grant for $98,000 to facilitate this process, we are working to ensure we do so in a *just* manner. As Ageyman (2013: 71) recognizes, "Producing and consuming locally does not guarantee any greater concern for social justice or more ecologically sustainable practices unless those principles are internalized into the movement," or in this case into CLiCK's practices.

In focusing on local food CLiCK is part of the "alternative food" movements which Alison Hope Alkon and Julian Agyeman describe in *Cultivating Food Justice* (2011: 1) as having "… crafted strong and coherent opposition to … industrial monoculture … [that] favors large farms with available capital, and have led to increased consolidation and corporate ownership of agriculture … [and which is] environmentally harmful." Therefore, for most of these food-based movements consumers/customers have come to recognize what they eat is not just a personal choice but is in fact a political act regardless of whether we see it as such. Hence, such slogans as "eat organic" or "shop local" or "Yes Farms, Yes Food" have become emblematic for many. Nevertheless, as with the emphases on local, what is not often addressed are the social and economic structures that make the "faces" behind these slogans appear homogeneous – as in being for the most part white and upper-middle class. This is not to say that they are in fact homogeneous. There are many branches of the food movement that are led by people of color, including Growing Power in Detroit, the Black Farmers Coalition, and La Via Compesina, discussed below. However, it is to acknowledge that questioning and analyzing issues of race, class and gender have been marginalized. Thus, as with Agyeman's emphasis on "*just* sustainabilities," CLiCK is influenced by the notion of "food justice" that sees direct links between social justice (economic and social equity) and food, as in both "food access" and "food sovereignty." Food access is based on people's ability to grow and or consume healthy food. Food sovereignty, as defined by the international farmers' activist group La Via Campesina, is a community's "right to define their own food and agriculture systems" (Via Campesina 2002).

Examples of how CLiCK has embodied these ideas are: choosing to be a non-profit as opposed to for-profit; being membership-based so that members have a voice in how CLiCK is organized; building a shared-use space so members are empowered to produce food products for themselves thereby enhancing the local economy; building a teaching kitchen where community members can learn healthy cooking; being committed to bilingualism so that all in the community can access information; creating community gardens and an orchard to enable community members to experience growing their own food; and holding culturally specific food festivals to reflect the diversity of the community (e.g. CLiCK's Salsa and Coquito Festivals). CLiCK therefore recognizes that just as personal food choices are political, so are the choices made by institutions as to how they are organized, their priorities, and how they conduct their affairs.

CLiCK is governed by a Board of Directors representing a diverse demographic in terms of social class, education, profession, experience, sex / sexuality and nationality. There is a deficit on CLiCK's Board in terms of racial / ethnic diversity, which is not uncommon for non-profits. Environmentalist Dorceta Taylor (2014) surveyed 191 environmental non-profits and found a significant lack of diversity, in particular when it comes to Board slots with on average only 4.6 percent held by people of color. Such a deficit is ironic given that people of color support the goals of environmental protection at higher rates than do whites. One barrier CLiCK has found is that those Latinos who would like to serve are prevented from doing so due to work and family commitments, which speaks to the issues of economic, social and racial inequality in the larger society that then get reflected in who has the time and the resources to serve. This is not an excuse but rather a social analysis of the conditions that help create the situation for CLiCK and likely for other organizations. In contrast to the finding that "efforts to attract and retain talented people of color have been lackluster" (http://diversegreen. org/report/ 2014), CLiCK is pursuing targeted outreach to qualified and interested members of the Latino community, itself broadly defined and very diverse. In addition, CLiCK is working closely with many members of the Latino community who either want to use the kitchen space to incubate their businesses, or who want to offer health and nutrition classes in the teaching kitchen.

By claiming that CLiCK is trying to put the concepts of "just sustainabilities" and "food justice" into practice by offering kitchens as a form of the commons, I have attempted to provide sufficient support so that readers can make their own judgments.

In addition, my emphasis on "social justice" is supported by many but not all members of the CLiCK Board. We have had some struggles over whether issues of "social justice" are a divergence from our "real mission" to provide a commercial kitchen and to generate income allowing self-sufficiency. However, I have asserted repeatedly that without such an emphasis we have nothing to offer that is new ideologically and in practice, and without that it cannot make the kind of changes we need as a community and as a society. This ongoing engagement has, I think, borne fruit as I recently heard one of these more skeptical Board members enthusiastically telling a possible funder that "CLiCK is a philosophy" – with which I couldn't agree more. It's a philosophy that recognizes the "means" must match "ends" and that both must be based on collective justice that begins with a common commitment for access to healthy, affordable and preferably local food.

Hedley Freake: perspectives of a nutritional scientist

I became aware of the nascent CLiCK in 2010. I had just returned from a year living in Hong Kong and thus was viewing the U.S. food systems, as specifically evidenced in rural northeastern Connecticut, with new perspectives informed by that experience. Hong Kong is a large, densely populated and very modern city. However, people's attitudes towards and expectations of food are grounded in centuries of tradition. In the U.S., we hear a lot about pollution in China and lack of safety in the food supply chain. These are real issues, that are somewhat mitigated in the politically and economically distinct circumstances of the Special Administrative Region of Hong Kong, in comparison to the mainland.

However, we don't hear about the wet markets, found in every neighborhood, where people shop daily, selecting from an abundance of fresh vegetables and fruits, live fish, pork and chicken. We do not know about the increasing number of small organic farms, located in the rural New Territories of Hong Kong, where farmers are following traditional methods and supplying produce that is trusted more than that brought in from the mainland. Hong Kong has many affordable restaurants that serve fresh, tasty and nutritious food. It is also the home of a myriad of small (and not so small) food processing operations. Everything from tofu and soy sauce to dried mushrooms, dried shrimp paste and XO sauce. Indeed, food processing in Hong Kong is designed to preserve the nutritional value and flavor of the raw ingredients, rather than develop novel products that dazzle the sensibilities of the consumer and enhance the market share of the manufacturer. There are many other dimensions to these contrasts between the food systems of Hong Kong and those of the United States (Freake 2014) but the end result is a food supply in Hong Kong that is fresh, less processed, locally derived and affordable.

The desire to stimulate a local food system with greater similarities to that of Hong Kong was one strand that provoked my involvement with CLiCK. Another was to better integrate my role as a Professor of Nutritional Sciences at the University of Connecticut with that of a citizen of my local community. Connecticut is, on average, a very wealthy state. But that average conceals great disparities that can be seen with respect to income, educational achievement and health outcomes. As stated above, Willimantic and Windham represent the disadvantaged portions of the state. The main campus of the University of Connecticut in Storrs is less than 10 miles away, but on another planet in the minds of many of its students. Limited public transportation does not help, but many of them spend 4 years completing their degrees and never get into Willimantic. This is partly ignorance – they are simply unaware of what the town has to offer. But it is also intentional avoidance based on misinformation – they have heard that it is unsafe, with a drug culture associated with its Latino population. Parenthetically, it could be pointed out that drug problems are at least as great in high schools located in wealthy white communities. Students at Windham High School don't have the resources to support a drug habit.

While Community Outreach programs based at the University do target Willimantic, the number of students involved is limited. In its first year of operation, CLiCK benefited from teams of UConn students who helped in the renovation and preparation of its space. One student obtained funding from the University to develop vegetable gardens in the grounds adjacent to the CLiCK building. The goal is to operate them in association with groups working with at-risk populations in Willimantic. In addition, a small number of students from nutrition and other disciplines have been excited by the CLiCK vision and have been working with its General Manager on getting the commercial kitchen set up and developing materials to attract members. Part of the model for setting up the teaching kitchen is to include nutrition students in the delivery of services to the local community. Their training as nutrition professionals needs to include the issues associated with "just sustainabilities" and "food justice" discussed above. While students bring nutrition expertise, at CLiCK they will be drawn into a model that first requires them to listen to and learn from community members, who will define the important issues and the help they are seeking.

Community-based research, two-way sharing of expertise and delivery of services are an integral part of the land grant mission of the University and in particular of the College of Agriculture, Health and Natural Resources, that contains Nutritional Sciences. This includes the federal Expanded Food and Nutrition Education Program that provides classes for low-income families. This established program will benefit from the facilities associated with the teaching kitchen that enable a much more hands-on approach to learning about preparing healthy food. A central part of the teaching kitchen philosophy is that of learning by doing and having local people be directly introduced to foods and approaches to preparing them that may be unfamiliar. Giving people the opportunity to prepare dishes themselves and then to share them with their families is more likely to lead to sustainable change in eating habits.

The community in which CLiCK is embedded suffers from high rates of both food insecurity and obesity. The coexistence of these two conditions is well established and focus is now on identifying the mediators that connect them (see Franklin et al. 2012). For example, food insecurity may lead to consumption of easily available inexpensive foods that are energy dense but nutrient poor. The health risks associated with obesity include increased incidence of Type-2

Diabetes (T2D) and cardiovascular diseases. The CLiCK model is constructed to address these issues on multiple levels. Nutrition education classes will assist individuals with T2D to better manage their disease by learning to cook foods that have less deleterious effects on the glycemic response. Those classes will be experiential in nature so that participants will learn how to prepare unfamiliar foods and familiar foods in different ways. The practical learning is more likely to lead to behavior change and positive health outcomes (Archuleta et al. 2012).

In addition to working to change the behaviors of individuals taking the classes, the intent is that CLiCK will impact the local food economy in larger ways. The commercial kitchen has begun to provide opportunities to farmers and other local people to enhance their livelihoods by developing food related businesses. Increasing economic security is likely to lead to decreased food insecurity. In addition, greater availability of locally produced foods will provide more alternatives to the nutrient-poor offerings currently consumed. CLiCK believes that a local food system that supports both the economic livelihood and the health of community members can be developed.

It is important that the field of nutrition and the education of nutrition students be conceptualized broadly to consider issues beyond the biochemical function of nutrients and their effects on the health of individuals. Dietary patterns, rather than individual nutrients and foods, are important and so are considerations of how food is grown, prepared and consumed. For 50 years now, the Mediterranean Diet has been associated with favorable health outcomes, but recent conceptualizations of this diet have moved beyond considering the foods that it contains (Bach-Faig et al. 2011). The food list is quite variable, depending on country, though an emphasis on fresh fruits and vegetables is common. The base of the Mediterranean Diet Pyramid, designed to give public recommendations about approaches to eating, includes "Culinary Activities" and "Conviviality." Care is to be taken in the preparation of meals and then time spent eating them with friends and family. "Biodiversity and seasonality" and "Traditional, local and eco-friendly products" are also listed as important elements. In the United States, commercialization, globalization and farm policies result in a food supply that is far from fresh and local. Social and economic pressures mitigate against people taking the time to cook and eat together. The agricultural system, with an emphasis on a small number of commodity crops and industrial animal production, is far from eco-friendly.

This broader conceptualization is quite consistent with Agyeman's "just sustainabilities." Nutrition is directed towards improving quality of life and well-being. But the quality of everybody's life needs to be considered and so food disparities within and between countries are of vital importance. The needs of future generations demand sustainable agricultural systems, rather than simply nutritious and tasty foods flown in from the other side of the world. As we think about the foods we consume, we need to take into account the treatment and rights of the people who were involved in growing and processing that food. Cheap food for us often comes at a cost to those who produce it.

Moving nutrition beyond nutrients leads to the concept of "just nutrition," where issues of social class, racism, and gender are understood as important elements that influence food access and nutritional outcomes. These same elements are, of course, important predictors of health outcomes, such as diabetes, cardiovascular disease and cancer via pathways that are both nutrition-dependent (overconsumption of cheap and filling foods of limited nutritional value) and independent (stress, access to health care).

CLiCK is envisaged as a venue that supports the economic, physical and social health of its communities with an emphasis on "just nutrition." Thus, food entrepreneurs using the commercial kitchens are encouraged to consider the nutritional benefits associated with their products along with the sourcing of their ingredients. Classes in the teaching kitchen particularly target at-risk and underserved populations, utilizing grant funds to underwrite their costs. Other educational and cultural activities focused on food will be put in a context that considers relevant social, cultural and ecological factors. Educational and outreach activities will be directed in a way that seeks to empower local people with the knowledge and skills required for improving their nutritional health. Thus CLiCK is not only part of a physical commons providing shared commercial kitchen space but also of the knowledge commons, creating a repository of shared food practices that can benefit the whole community.

Challenges moving forward

CLiCK is a very young organization. Nevertheless, it already has enjoyed significant successes, facilitating the creation of new businesses and acting as a focus for community food and nutrition education efforts.

But we face significant challenges that we are struggling to address as the project moves forward. The largest of these is probably financial. Despite considerable success in attracting approximately $300,000 in grant funds, CLiCK is significantly undercapitalized and is located in an undercapitalized section of Connecticut. The renovations to create the kitchens ran over budget, primarily because of unforeseen (and perhaps unforeseeable) additional costs. Thus there is a capital improvement deficit that needs to be addressed. The business model for CLiCK is that membership dues and kitchen usage fees are sufficient in aggregate to pay the running costs of the business, including manager salary, utility bills, cost of consumables, etc. However, it takes time for those revenue streams to build. The manager salary can and will for the foreseeable future be paid from grant funds. However, most grant sources will not pay for the basic operating costs of the building and until kitchen usage builds to match these expenses, we are operating at a deficit. This situation is faced by every new business and so is not unexpected but still needs to be addressed.

A similar 501(c)(3) non-profit kitchen project is CommonWealth Kitchen in Boston, whose mission is "to strengthen the local economy, particularly for people who have been impacted by racial, social, and economic inequality" (http://www.commonwealthkitchen.org). However, as already noted, CommonWealth does not offer nutrition or culinary education, nor is there a particular emphasis on processing or using locally grown products. Additionally, it is a much larger operation and is located in a large city where access to resources and entrepreneurs is much greater. Even with these advantages, CommonWealth still gets 60 percent of its income from grants and donations, indicating that CLiCK will likewise need to continue seeking grants and donations to serve its mission. Grants are obtainable for developing programs both for local food business development and nutrition education, but unrestricted funds that can be used to support operating costs are required. These applications are being written, but the sources available are more limited in rural northeast Connecticut than in other locales. The same is true for community fund-raising. CLiCK is sited where the needs are greatest and wealthy local donors are scarcest.

CLiCK is focused on creating pathways between the local production of raw fruits and vegetables by small-scale farmers and the marginal market demand for locally processed food products. On a large scale this pathway between farm, processing and consumer is easily handled by global food corporations that buy in massive amounts from industrialized mono-cropping farms that then process a product for the purpose of turning a large profit once the product is finally purchased (Patel 2012). This can be illustrated by looking at the differences between the prices of raw fruits and vegetables versus the products that they become once processed. For example, potato chips cost 100 times more than the potatoes from which they are made. Hence, what CLiCK is trying to do is to move the food from one local actor (the farmer), to another local actor (CLiCK), to the final local actor (the consumer) while simultaneously enabling all to benefit in ways that embody "just sustainability."

However, the pathways are not set up to make this people-to-people movement an easy endeavor. The options in place for small-scale local farmers are to sell their raw goods at farmers markets or through CSAs and / or to leave any processing either to their own very small-scale endeavors or to the big farms. Likewise, for CLiCK the options in place are to have enough capital to buy raw fruits and vegetables in bulk and to then focus on processing for a profit, as opposed to for the collective, common good in terms of increasing the availability of locally processed foods. Currently, CLiCK does not have the capital to buy fruits and vegetables to create this local stream. Even when such programs are grant funded, the funding model is one of reimbursement, so up-front cash is needed to start the process. For the customer, the options in place are to buy locally grown raw fruits or vegetables, or to buy processed ones that have been grown, processed, packaged, shipped, marketed and sold for the purpose of profiting large food corporations. Thus, the fact that CLiCK is struggling in terms of how to process locally grown foods, even on a small scale, should not be surprising as we are swimming against the corporate tide. We are trying to create economic and social pathways on a local scale that connect people to people along the chains of supply and demand with the objective being something other than profit.

One adjustment to the original model that has been required results from the fact that farmers do not have the time to process and add value to their fruits and vegetables themselves. They are happy to sell what they grow to CLiCK and have other CLiCK members or staff do the work, though again this requires initial capital to get the process running. The first CLiCK kitchen members who are developing their own businesses have been doing this partially and it is anticipated this will continue to build as we attract new members and build relationships between farmers and food entrepreneurs.

Early members are also generally white and tend to come from well-educated middle class backgrounds with the resources, knowledge and self-confidence to develop a new business. Extensive outreach efforts to less privileged community members are ongoing and have yielded expressions of interest. The kitchen manager is working with a number of these individuals to develop business plans and share the knowledge required. Still, financial considerations make it difficult for these individuals, just as it does for CLiCK itself. One solution is to pursue grant funds that can be used to subsidize the start-up costs as these people work to develop their new business. In fact, CLiCK has recently applied for two such grants and has plans to apply to others to further ensure we are putting our commitments into practice.

CLiCK continues to deal with these challenges using a process that reaches out as broadly as possible to its community and particularly those parts of it that share common interests. Local "institutions" like the Willimantic Food Co-op and the No Freeze Shelter (for the homeless) are well grounded in our community, experienced at fund-raising and generating community support, and absolutely supportive of CLiCK and its mission. Importantly, we understand that we develop strength and effectiveness by working together.

Conclusion: linking theory and practice

One of the most fascinating aspects of working on and with CLiCK for both of us has been to watch aspects of our academic disciplines as "theories" come into being as practices and as members of the Board to further guide and revise those theories as new issues emerge and new practices are needed. Our current financial challenges, in the case of a for-profit business, might indicate a fault with the overall model in terms of the business's ability to create enough profit to sustain itself. However, in CLiCK's case our model of seeking to support small-scale farmers though local processing, small food business creation and health and nutrition education is not the problem, and is in fact the solution for so many of our social, economic and health based problems. The *problem* is the larger industrial food system that like Goliath has a great advantage over David, especially a very small and recently established David, and therefore makes creating even a small change challenging. Regardless, what CLiCK has on its side, like the original David, is righteousness in terms of not only speaking about a more just, equitable, sustainable, held in common, food system but more audaciously of trying to create one.

In this manner CLiCK is a social and economic experiment whose success or failure doesn't just depend on our individual efforts but rather on the larger questions as to whether we as a community and as a society are committed to change our local and national food systems to serve the interests of all life as opposed to the corporate interests of a few. It is too soon to know the answer for CLiCK or for the larger society but we feel that there is a better chance of the answer being "Yes" if more communities follow CLiCK's lead. CLiCK offers a theoretical model based on "just sustainabilities" and "just nutrition" that encourages community control over "the commons," be that a kitchen, knowledge, land, food, or anything else essential to the well-being of a community. Additionally, CLiCK offers a practical model in terms of what these theories can look like at a grassroots level while allowing for variability to suit the specific social, economic and geographic locations. An increasing demand for local food, coupled with greater public awareness of the importance of environmental issues, including climate change and the continuing roles that racism and poverty play in the United States make us optimistic. The time is right for CLiCK and other initiatives like it that incorporate understanding of these issues in their mission and make them central to their daily practices.

References

Agyeman, J. 2003. *Just Sustainabilities: Development in an Unequal World.* Cambridge, MA: MIT Press.

Agyeman, J. 2013. *Introducing Just Sustainabilities: Policy, Planning and Practices.* New York: Zed Books.

Alkon, A., and Agyeman, J. 2011. *Cultivating Food Justice: Race, Class and Sustainability.* Cambridge, MA: MIT Press.

Archuleta, M.L, Vanleeuwen, D., Halderson, K., Jackson, K., Bock, M.A., Eastman, W., Powell, J., Titone, M., Marr, C., and Wells, L. 2012. "Cooking schools improve nutrient intake patterns of people with type 2 diabetes." *J Nutr Educ Behav.* 44(4): 319–325.

Bach-Faig, A., Berry, E.M., Lairon, D., Reguant, J., Trichopoulou, A., Dernini, S., Medina, F.X., Battino, M., Belahsen, R., Miranda, G., and Serra-Majem, L. (Mediterranean Diet Foundation Expert Group) 2011. "Mediterranean diet pyramid today: Science and cultural updates." *Public Health Nutr.* 14(12A): 2274–2284.

CLiCK n.d. CLiCK website. Available online at http://clickwillimantic.com/ (accessed May 25, 2016).

Cox, M., Arnold, G., and Villamayor Tomás, S. 2010. "A review of design principles for community-based natural resource management." *Ecology and Society* 15(4): 38. Available online at http://www.ecologyandsociety.org/vol15/iss4/art38/ (accessed November 23, 2015).

Felice, F. and Vatiero, M. 2012. "Elinor Ostrom and the solution to the tragedy of the commons." *Il Sussidiario*, June 27. Available online at www.aei.org/publication/elinor-ostrom-and-the-solution-to-the-tragedy-of-the-commons/ (accessed November 23, 2015).

Franklin, B., Jones, A., Love, D., Puckett, S., Macklin, J., and White-Means, S. 2012. "Exploring mediators of food insecurity and obesity: A review of recent literature." *J Community Health* 37: 253–264.

Freake, H. 2014. *Eating Hong Kong.* In J. Curry and P. Hanstedt (eds.), *Reading Hong Kong, Reading Ourselves.* Hong Kong: City University of Hong Kong Press.

Hardin, G. 1968. "The tragedy of the commons." *Science* 162: 1243–1248.

Hinrichs, C.C., and Lyson, T.A. 2007. *Remaking the North American Food System: Strategies for Sustainability.* Cambridge, MA: MIT Press.

Moyer, J. 2015. *What Nobody Told Me about Small Farming: I Can't Make a Living.* Available online at www.salon.com/2015/02/10/what_nobody_told_me_about_small_farming_i_cant_make_a_living/ (accessed November 23, 2015).

Patel, R. 2012. *Stuffed and Starved: The Hidden Battle for the World Food System* (Revised and updated). New York: Melville House.

Ostrom, E. 1990. *Governing the Commons: The Evolution of Institutions for Collective Action.* Cambridge: Cambridge University Press.

Ostrom, E., Burger, J., Field, C.B., Norgaard, R.B., and Policansky, D. 1999. "Revisiting the commons: Local lessons, global challenges." *Science* 284: 278–282.

Taylor, D. 2014. *The State of Diversity in Environmental Organizations: Mainstream NGOs, Foundations & Government Agencies.* Available online at http://diversegreen.org/report/ (accessed March 17, 2015).

9 Developing a food system-sensitive methodology to transform food "waste," create new food businesses, and address hunger in urban communities

Thomas H. O'Donnell, Jonathan Deutsch, Cathy Yungmann, Alexandra Zeitz, and Solomon H. Katz

Over the eight years since the onset of the great food crisis of 2007–09, when high food prices forced over 200 million additional people into the ranks of the hungry, global humanity crossed a new threshold with well over a billion people in hunger. This realization has forced new and important considerations about our capacity to feed a world population expected to be about 9.6 billion by 2050 even as very serious climate-change effects threaten to decrease the current productivity of our agricultural system.

A similarly severe food crisis occurred in the early 1970s, when lower crop productivity could not keep up with demand, and soaring food prices resulted in additional millions being forced into hunger. However, in that earlier case, the "Green Revolution" replaced traditional agricultural methods with new hybridized seed and agricultural practices that, among others, used extensive irrigation to maintain cereal grains through critical water-sensitive periods of early growth to maintain high productivity. Whether a similar technological revolution can stave off global hunger by mid-century is problematic. For example, crop productivity is decreasing as irrigation has been over-used and ground water aquifers in many parts of the world are severely reduced or depleted.

The deeply worrisome added conditions of climate change impacting food production at rates and magnitudes of change that have never been encountered will need to be balanced by new measures and a focus on the entire food system. The announcement of the United Nations Sustainable Development Goals in 2015 offers some hope in this regard, with the Sustainable Development Goal #12, Target 12.3, focusing on cutting consumer and retail food waste by 50 percent by the year 2030, while reducing food loss along the production and supply chain (Sustainable Development, n.d.). However, in the midst of these new global initiatives, a new and very promising perspective about making better use of food that is already produced is quickly developing; in September 2015, the United States Environmental Protection Agency (EPA) and United States Department of Agriculture announced a new goal to halve US food waste by 2030 (USDA(a) n.d.; USEPA(a) n.d.). The issue is simple and the possibilities for quick action that could multiply the potentials of food already available are enormous.

Wasted food is a grossly overlooked resource that stands in easy reach for overcoming some of our far too prevalent hunger. Widespread, active participation in eliminating food waste could relieve this problem in a relatively short time – potentially much quicker, in fact, than current attempts to increase field productivity. Indeed, minimizing food waste could extend current global output of food production by at least 15 percent in a matter of less than a decade. Better and more complete utilization of food resources already being produced also means lessening the environmental resources needed to produce more food. This will mean that for every unit of food saved, there will be substantially less new need for water, land use, fertilizers, pesticides and herbicides. Finally, given the immense amount of food that ends up in landfills, producing methane, reducing food waste also can contribute to a substantial decrease in greenhouse gas emissions.

Waste occurs everywhere in the food system. However, there are some opportunities for addressing waste at points in the food chain where substantial increases in efficiency can be achieved. This chapter presents several "downstream" innovations that are being evaluated as new methods to create food products from supermarket produce that is otherwise just thrown away. The idea is to convert nutritious fruits and vegetables that a grocer decides to remove from the sales aisle into new kinds of products packaged for resale or inputs for food service and restaurant offerings. Preliminary analysis indicates that by maintaining low input costs from food that would otherwise be donated or disposed and by using few added ingredients, new products can be made and sold at an affordable price point. Pricing fruits and vegetables at more favorable levels using limited processing is promising in encouraging more consumption of these important components of the Dietary Guidelines for Americans (Health.gov n.d.). This chapter provides insight into the health and economic benefits available through this methodology. New ways to educate others on the process is also presented with the intent of helping to build a scalable method that other areas can replicate.

Surplus food and urban hunger

The number of people living in cities with populations over 30,000 who experience hunger and ask for help continued to increase in 2014 (Chokshi 2014). According to the U.S. Conference of Mayors (2014), 72 percent of cities surveyed reported increased requests for food assistance. Over half of these were families and over a third of the adults were working. Importantly for the innovations described in this chapter, over a quarter of the requests for food assistance went unmet. With 48 million Americans reporting food insecurity in 2014, emergency food distribution systems cannot keep up with demand even as more and more people are malnourished, as indicated by increasing obesity rates among SNAP recipients seeking cheap and filling but unhealthy options (USDA, FNS n.d.). In fact, in 82 percent of the cities surveyed by the Conference, emergency food kitchens and pantries *reduced* the quantity of food reaching people in need, a divergence between need and capacity that is projected to continue. Providing more jobs and more training were cited by two-thirds of the cities as key remedies for their hunger problems. New jobs and training are also key outcomes of the program described here.

These trends reflect on the solutions that have been used to try and put a practical end to food insecurity. For decades, hunger has been addressed by government programs, particularly the Supplemental Nutrition Assistance Program (SNAP), formerly known as food stamps (USDA(b) n.d.), and the thousands of hunger relief, charitable organizations that distribute to people in local communities (Feeding America n.d.). New efforts to reduce the amount of environmentally damaging food waste by feeding people in need have also contributed to the solution. The EPA and USDA both have an interest in shifting the food waste problem toward beneficial uses (USEPA(a) n.d., USDA(c) n.d.). States and municipalities have responded by imposing food waste disposal bans (Massachusetts n.d.; SFEnvironment n.d.). One pillar of sustainable food management, economics, holds great potential for innovations to reduce hunger while leveraging new jobs and business opportunities (Figure 9.1). For example, a focus on converting surplus food to new products links powerful economic drivers to the highest tier of the EPA's Food Recovery Challenge, which is food waste prevention or source reduction.

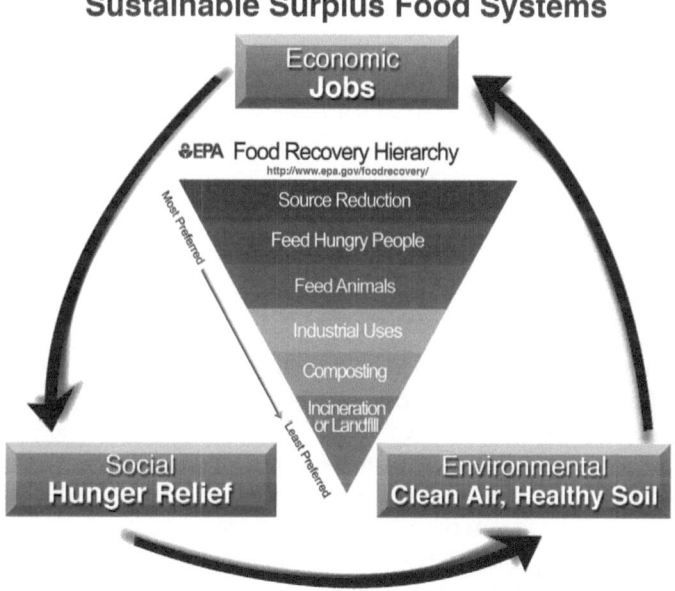

Figure 9.1   Sustainable Surplus food systems

Opportunities for surplus food

Gunders (2012) reported that more than half of the wasted food in the United States occurs at the consumer level. Of that portion, about half of this food was wasted by households, while the rest came from restaurants and grocery stores. The Grocery Manufacturers Association and Food Marketing Institute surveyed their industries and found that although most food waste occurs from residences and food service, a significant amount comes from grocery stores. This chapter focuses on waste at the retail level with a full acknowledgement that there is waste in the entire system.

Downstream, in the consumer space, fruits and vegetables lead the food waste category, followed closely by dairy, meat and seafood. Each of these has one or more beneficial use options within the Food Recovery Hierarchy. Composting, for example, is a proven way to use household and restaurant food waste. Industrial organizations are often able to recycle their food waste or feed it to animals. Grocery stores and the distributors that supply them are unique in having food that is packaged, delivered, and marketed for direct consumption. Some supermarkets have a track record of using in-house products, such as dairy, produce, and bakery, to prepare foods for their deli section, salad bars, and take-out meals, while others cite expensive labor, lack of equipment and lack of trained staff as obstacles to in-store food conversion. In some instances, foods are converted into packaged, value-added products to extend their lives in new appealing ways for customers to buy.

As such, supermarkets provide an obvious place to evaluate new uses for food about to be put into the waste system. Customer-facing produce for example, the primary subject of our current research, is inspected at least daily by trained store personnel whose job it is to be sure their freshest products are displayed. Much of the produce that is removed from the aisles for disposal may be ripe or overripe, have cosmetic defects, or otherwise not be the best available. It is almost always still usable and just as nutritious – sometimes more due to ripeness - as before it was taken off the shelf. The quantity of this sort of product on a regional scale is very large. The EPA reports that 113.7 million pounds of produce was wasted in 2010 (WARM 2015). Gunders (2012) reports that produce constitutes 22 percent of the food waste stream. Millions of tons of food are wasted each year and a significant source with high potential revenue value comes from the more than 37,000 large supermarkets in the United States (FMI n.d.). The fact that these sources are numerous and situated in many communities with a need for hunger relief, jobs, and new businesses encouraged the evaluation in this chapter.

New programs to use fruits and vegetables that have not traditionally been accepted in stores or food service due to arbitrary cosmetic standards are sprouting in Europe, Canada, and the United States. This expanded avenue for delivering bulk produce to consumers has the potential to significantly reduce farm and processing-level food loss. North American distributor programs with names like Misfits (Shelby Report 2015) or Imperfect Produce (n.d.) work with farmers to move these products to their retail and wholesale distributors. With direct connection to farms and grocers, the food distributors also add to promotional marketing, sales, and information technology support. Although the farmers absorb the impact of lower prices, grocers need to be certain that selling produce at 30 percent discounts or more can increase sales volume overall to justify dedicated floor space. Supermarkets are running promotions of these products with names like "Real Good produce" (NPR 2015) or "Misfits" (Robinson Fresh n.d.). Food service companies are grasping the opportunity as well. Compass Group's "ImperfectVeg" program (Church Brothers n.d.) and Bon Appetit's "Imperfectly Delicious" Produce (BAMCO n.d.) are sourcing "seconds" from farmers and wholesale distributors for their kitchens where chefs can work with food that may not be ideal for grocery stores (SFGate 2015). Hunger relief organizations seeing the potential for healthy produce at bulk costs are learning to recovery and process food in their commercial kitchen and food processing facilities (L.A.Kitchen n.d.).

Food system-sensitive methodology (FSSM)

In 2015 our team (O'Donnell et al. 2015) reported on the organization of a new method for managing supermarket foods that are sent to waste management options listed in the Food Recovery Hierarchy (Figure 9.2). The Food System-

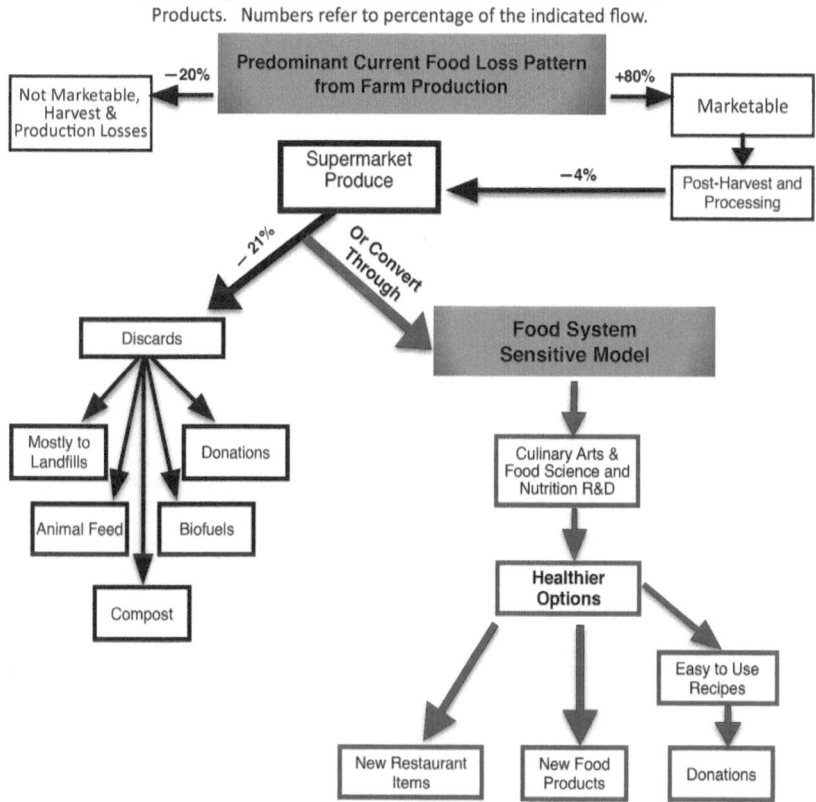

Figure 9.2 Life cycle of supermarket discards

Sensitive Methodology (FSSM) approach provides creative options to re-channel food from entering the waste management system at any level. The methodology improves the efficiency of the food system by converting food into new food products rather than categorizing it as food waste. The methodology also puts a high premium on healthy food options that are preferred by most consumers, which is accomplished by utilizing the skills afforded by culinary arts, food science, nutrition, and public health.

Currently, new food options are being tested for two economic options, food products and restaurant menu options, and two social outcomes, hunger relief and social entrepreneurship. In this manner, FSSM supports tools to eliminate the causes of food insecurity by identifying new business and job opportunities while also continuing to support the ongoing needs of people who need a daily meal. It is this management focus on food insecurity eradication and the health and education for participants that defines the current use of the system-sensitive modality.

Developing a case study

The food system is everywhere complex, so any investigation into new innovations must be supported by a skilled and committed team with similar goals and interests. These concepts are not new and can be applied in any community interested in local hunger relief. The case study inputs grew from analysis of parameters that would increase the likelihood of a successful pilot program and also allow continuous adaptation as new information and opportunities became apparent as it has. Different cities, towns, projects, and objectives will require different types of specialization. For this project we had a core group of organizations and support from experts listed in Table 9.1. These participants were supported and helped by the U.S. EPA and the USDA; The Enterprise Center, a local food manufacturing incubator; and various Philadelphia area hunger relief personnel and organizations. Underlying the individuals and groups was a vision for local food sourcing and jobs, community networks, local media communications, healthy neighborhoods, and a view towards zero waste.

Table 9.1 Subject matter expertise and resource groups for the pilot project

Subject matter experts	Resources, organizations, and specialties
Culinary arts and food science	For profit food recycling businesses
Health and nutrition	Diverse sources of surplus food
Education	Food donation infrastructure
Supermarket management	Local composting systems
Food waste management	Social and environmental community aura
	Economic development district

Selection of a pilot project area

The initial stages of the project involved a planning study to identify key stakeholders to engage the community and determine the feasibility of such a project. Advisory Panel members included the Delaware Valley Planning Commission (DVRPC), Organic Diversion (a local composter), Philabundance (a local food bank), and the Bucks County Foodshed Alliance (a local food system NGO). Stakeholders determined that there was a need to explore new options for urban food recovery since the City of Philadelphia, where about 21 percent of residents are food insecure, represents some of the highest levels of food insecurity among large cities in America.

Utilizing a food Life Cycle Analysis (LCA) approach for the entire Philadelphia urban area, a geographic information system (GIS) database tool was developed to identify the largest generators of surplus food (hospitals, grocery, entertainment and sporting venues, universities, hotels, etc.) and possible receptors of surplus food (such as community gardens, food banks, and composting facilities). The West Philadelphia and University City neighborhoods in west Philadelphia were selected to implement the model based on a match to the criteria mentioned in the previous section, particularly having a rich diversity of surplus-food generators, local composting/donation facilities, a range of community gardens and urban farms, and a strong economic development improvement district.

University City is an approximately 2.4 square mile neighborhood in west Philadelphia that houses some of the best universities, hospitals, and transportation hubs in the City. It also is home to a large population of low-income residents who are supported by public and non-profit health and hunger relief organizations. Figure 9.3 shows the boundaries of University City and the Philadelphia Promise

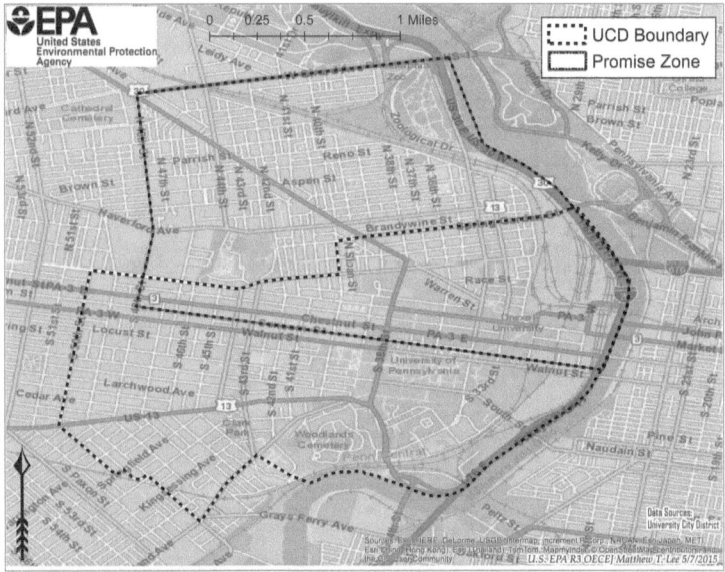

Figure 9.3   University City neighborhood

Zone designated by the federal government (HUD Exchange n.d.) as an area of investment focus for quality of life revitalization. The Urban Model for Surplus Food Recovery, a Region 3 EPA pilot, was initially launched in University City but expanded in collaboration with Drexel University once the Promise Zone designation was awarded.

University City lies within three ZIP codes and parts or all of 11 census tracts. The District shares its northern border with the Promise Zone. The eastern tracts of both are dominated by universities and hospitals; in the remaining areas are low-income communities with social and economic features similar to the rest of Philadelphia. Based on the most current census data for non-institutional portions of the area, 4,118 residents are food insecure (Table 9.2), in need of a consistent supply of affordable, nutritious food products but only having limited access or resources to buy them. Matching these food needs and supply limitations is one of the principal social drivers of our research. The pilot area is a testing ground to learn the degree to which surplus fresh foods from supermarkets can help meet some of the pricing and nutrient needs of lower income populations in this area and similar ones throughout the United States.

Feeding America, the nation's largest hunger relief organization, has created a concept and measurement tool referred to as the Meal Gap, which helps planners understand the magnitude of food insecurity in any county or congressional district in the United States (Feeding America n.d.). The tool can also be used in a general way to help understand the number and cost of additional meals on average that a community needs to close the Meal Gap, which is based on an estimate that food insecure people need 176 meals a year to satisfy minimum food requirements. In the project area, the number of additional meals needed per year is 724,768. Using the Feeding America weight of food per meal, this translates to 869,722 pounds of food. That is a large amount, but considering that a single

Table 9.2 Demographic characteristics in western UCD census tracts (78, 79, 80.01, 86.02, 91) and factors used to calculate a food insecurity rate

Factor	Value
Population	17,411
Food insecurity	24.1%
Food insecure population	4,118
Unemployment rate	6.7%
Poverty rate	26.0%
Median income	$30,159
Percent Black	27.0%
Percent Hispanic	4.7%
Percent own home	18.3%

Source: As calculated by Gundersen et al. 2013.

supermarket store disposes of as much or more than 50,000 pounds of food per year, it is not at all overwhelming. For example, that much wasted food may be recoverable from 17 grocery stores, not including the contribution of recovered surplus food from farming, food distribution, processing and manufacturing, or restaurants and food service. A considerable amount of the food may also be available through SNAP benefits.

Working with a supermarket

In March 2014, the EPA's Region 3, in partnership with Drexel University's Food Lab and Brown's Super Stores, a Philadelphia area supermarket chain, began to explore methods of converting culled, fresh produce from the stores into various fruit and vegetable product and meal items using creative recipes. The Drexel Food Lab, working with local community shelters and food cupboards, learned that much of the donated fresh produce was so fragile or undesirable to clients that it often was rejected before eaten, thereby diminishing the donation option and shifting waste and its cost from well-resourced retailers to struggling NGOs.

The concept of using culinary arts research and development to produce wholesome desirable foods free of any cosmetic issues evolved from these observations and the partnership. This is where the Food System-Sensitive Methodology emerged within the scope of the ongoing pilot project – one that recognized the possibility of avoiding food waste while using ripe nutritious surplus foods as inputs to new food products (Seymour et al. 2013). A working hypothesis also emerged that suggested that surplus food could be purchased at a reduced cost, thereby allowing products to be developed that could compete in the marketplace with unhealthy processed foods that were affordable and popular in underserved Philadelphia neighborhoods. Initial reports of this research were presented at various conferences while being popularized in blog posts (O'Donnell 2014; Lampert 2015), local news (Lazor 2014), and multi-media news organizations (Huffington Post 2015). The Federal Executive Board in May 2014 recognized the project as an example of *Outstanding Public Service* (FEB 2015), and in November 2014 the Administrator of the USEPA visited Philadelphia to laud the partners who were working to optimize the food transformation program (YouTube 2014).

Food research and development specialists from the Drexel University Culinary Arts and Food Science program are collaborating with Brown's Super Stores in Philadelphia to experiment with produce discards for the purpose of recipe and food product development. In April 2015, the 11 stores in the chain donated 68,039 pounds of food, of which 51.25 percent (34,870 pounds) was fresh fruits and vegetables. These products are a particular challenge due to their perishability. While meats, for example, are easily frozen before their sell-by day, kept in cold-storage and distributed to be defrosted and cooked by a social-service food provider, the same cannot be as easily done with produce.

The Drexel Food Lab's initial and ongoing 2015 surveys of discarded produce from a regional chain of stores found that approximately 25 percent was unusable/

trim such as moldy strawberries, brown greens, and bruised apples. Eliminating these components from the starting product weight left 26,152 pounds that was still useful for development (Figure 4). About 10 percent of the total was perfectly sound but specialty or unusual and not sufficient in quantity for production. For example, prickly pear cactus, kumquats, and avocados may be scattered in the mix of large quantities of sweet potatoes or kale. That reduced the practical yield to 22,665 pounds. By observation, if this remaining yield is served directly at a soup kitchen or shelter, fresh produce such as apples, baby carrot sticks, bananas, and oranges has about a 33 percent uptake. The remainder monthly amount, 15,185 pounds, was surplus food that could be used for new product development or prepared at a restaurant for retail customers. That amount of food was the starting base line that was used for thinking about new business opportunities and how creative social entrepreneurs can envision new products and solutions to the food waste challenge.

Although the sample pool was only one month from a single, 11-store chain, small relative to the amount of produce available for donation or product development throughout the year, and the sampling and analysis research is new, several preliminary results are available. The current Drexel Food Lab sustainable-market working model based on surplus food inputs from supermarkets is to purchase surplus food at a deep discount; for example, $.25 per pound or $8,717 in the example above. While not much revenue for a supermarket, this would be an additional revenue stream for what has formerly been a disposal expense. Continuing with this possible scenario, a social enterprise of community residents would process that surplus produce into value-added food products such as veggie chips, jams, smoothie bases and other products. These value-added products can then be wholesaled back to the same supermarket or other community-based retailers for $2.00 per pound. Accounting for the cost of added ingredients, labor

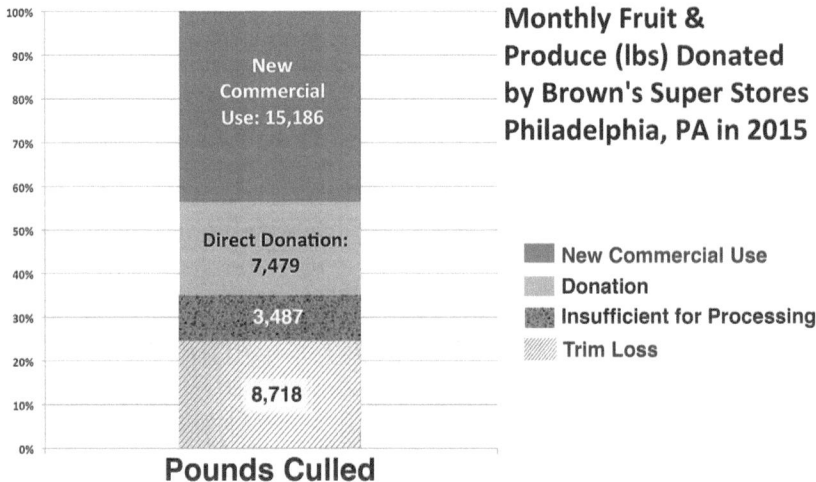

Figure 9.4   Monthly produce donated by Browns

and profit, generating up to $52,304 in monthly revenue (starting with 65 percent of monthly donated produce multiplied by two dollars per pound), and supporting two to four employees in new jobs at a family wage. These products can then be retailed at $3.99, generating $90,433 in monthly gross revenue for the store and $38,129 after cost of goods sold. The scalable economic, social, and environmental opportunities are potentially substantial.

Culinary arts, food science, and transforming surplus food

The actual recipe development and implementation for safe and cost-effective conversion of surplus food draws on the three prongs of the FSSM model that increases the nutritional quality and attractiveness of new recipes for foodservice, new food products, and easy to use recipes for hunger relief organizations. The Drexel Food Lab has three baskets of activities: product/recipe development and technical assistance for industry, good-food work for non-profits (pro-bono and grant funded), and the lab's own product development for technology transfer.

While definitions of "good food" vary widely with regard to sourcing, distribution, labor, health, nutrition and so on, one thing everyone in the good-food movement can agree on is that food should be eaten, not wasted. In this particular project, food lab students work with the EPA's Food Recovery Challenge in west Philadelphia to make sure that, once redistributed, surplus food is actually used.

An immediate question in discussing this work is typically whether the food converted is safe to eat. Food safety should be paramount in any food preparation. Even the finest restaurants have to deal with less-than-perfect products and cooks are trained to do so. It is important that cooks and managers be certified safe food handlers, such as through ServSafe certification from the National Restaurant Association or an equivalent, and learn which products can be safely repurposed, and how, and which need to be discarded. For example, bread that is moldy should be discarded; fruit that has a spot of mold may be trimmed and then cooked to a minimum temperature of 165 degrees Fahrenheit for at least 15 seconds, rather than being discarded.

In this research, the food lab started with the ingredients themselves from a culinary perspective. Imagine something like wrinkled grape tomatoes, for example. What can be done with them that will require few special skills and few added ingredients to make them appealing? We know what *won't* work is to serve them as is—they do not look appetizing. How can we best take advantage of the food—sweet ripeness, stunning red color, good bite? We might toss them with herbs and do an oven-dry; cook them for jam, sauce, or condiment; a lightly cooked pickle; a leather or granita. There are numerous possibilities, but it all starts with highlighting the best possibilities of the food and being careful to limit additional costs.

In this work, health is important. Most of the foods being identified as surplus at the retail level are fresh fruits and vegetables, which tend to be nutritionally dense and not very caloric. The Drexel Food Lab also lives by the premise that in general, the healthiest foods are scratch-cooked. The primary goal is to make the food delicious and eaten rather than composted or landfilled. We are not strictly developing food for weight loss or particular health states like diabetes but rather trying to give a new life to foods destined for the compost or landfill. It remains up to individual consumers to eat the types and amounts of foods right for them if they can afford that luxury of choice.

The next step in this process is to work with a commercial kitchen to scale-up and commercialize these foods. We believe there could be a model to purchase surplus foods at a discount, add value, and resell them as wholesale or retail products. The strongest model is one where a business can make the process work, as there will be real incentive through a market-driven problem-solving approach. This idea then builds on the economic pillar of sustainability, which has not been sufficiently developed.

The Drexel Food Lab is expanding this model to a community café in West Philadelphia, the Eat Café (n.d.) that will have surplus food as its primary food source. The concept here is to provide meals using ripe produce that can be offered at a range of prices so everyone in a community can enjoy delicious food at a price they can afford. Doing so requires a talented and flexible chef and good team of cooks. The cost benefits of converting foods that would previously go towards recycling or waste is the driver for this concept. Blue Hill Restaurant (Schwaner-Albright 2015) and others (The Real Junk Food Project n.d.) have engaged in this concept and demonstrated some ways it can work.

One key to success is to process the food immediately upon receipt. Often we are working with food that a food bank will not accept because the few days of the distribution cycle would do too much damage to the food. We only receive surplus food on the day when we have capacity to cook it. Foods are immediately washed and trimmed. If we have excess we can pickle, can, freeze or otherwise preserve before the next culinary application. For example, brown bananas are immediately peeled, pureed and frozen and then can be used in a wide variety of applications: smoothies, "ice creams," and so on. This takes extra labor, so the surplus food must be available at a deep discount if we are talking about commercializing.

To give a sense of the variety and quantity of products culled from supermarket shelves and developed into recipes for this project, Table 9.3 represents typical daily quantities (in pounds unless otherwise specified) of culled products for Drexel Food Lab R&D.

As the rare research university with a culinary degree program in the United States, the lab has a special obligation not only to teach people how to cook but also to apply their culinary skills to real world problems. Our next project needs to be a way to disseminate our ideas and provide support, the topic of the next section. This is not a local problem. The foods we pick up locally are the same, with some variation, coming into soup kitchen and shelter doors around the country. A web-repository with multi-lingual video recipes is the plan as well as turnkey templates for social enterprises that can convert these foods.

Preliminary analyses of the scalable and reproducible outcomes for these ideas have been published by O'Donnell et al. (2015a, 2015b). One scenario showed

Table 9.3 Examples of Drexel Food Lab conversions of surplus fruits and vegetables into products and recipes

Food type	Weight as received (pounds unless otherwise noted)	Usable for conversion	Product development
Green grapes	48.1	32.1	Drying
Grapes – red and green	22.6	22.6	Preserves
Blueberries	7.2	4.5	Baking
Bell peppers – red, yellow, orange	17.8	13.8	Roast and jar
Oranges	78.3	47.2	Juice
Tomatoes	11.1	11.1	Oven dry
Tomatoes	5.3	4.3	Sauce
Grape tomatoes	3 boxes	3 boxes	Oven dry
Pears	6.5	6.5	Juice
Apples	28.4	21.7	Juice
Mangoes	11.1	5.5	Juice
Lemons	3.5	3.0	Juice
Strawberries	13.0	9.7	Jam, preserves
Cantaloupes	33.6	33.6	Juice

how a single month's worth of surplus produce from Brown's Super Stores, an 11 store supermarket chain in Philadelphia, could be used to produce food products with potential gross revenue of nearly $40,000 for a social enterprise after deducting cost of goods sold. A noteworthy outcome of this demonstration was the scalable opportunities for new food product development for other groups that can access the billions of pounds of produce that supermarkets are not using. Another scenario looked at a more granular scale explaining how a one-month supply of culled tomatoes from one of the Brown's stores could be used to manufacture tomato jam. On a single day per week 700 pounds of tomatoes could be used to make 410 8-ounce jars of jam that could provide a gross profit to the social enterprise of $1,640 for the day's work. The scenarios are examples but both illustrate the possibilities for creating profitable social enterprise food businesses closely linked to the community. Other recipes and product testing like those mentioned in Table 9.3 are just the beginning.

Environmental benefits: greenhouse gases

Food waste (USEPA, 2016), paper, and yard trimmings create the bulk source of the 115.3 MMtCO2e of greenhouse gases released from landfills in 2012. At least half were from food waste, equivalent to emissions of 24,273,684 vehicles, annually.

The EPA created its Waste Reduction Model (USEPA, 2016.) to help people calculate the greenhouse gas emissions resulting from different waste management practices. The online software tool models fifty different types of materials and allows an estimate of food waste greenhouse gas (GHG) emissions from disposal

Table 9.4 GHG emissions resulting from 2012 landfill disposal of grains, fruits, and vegetables compared to waste prevention and from Brown's surplus food shown in Figure 9.4

Food group	Landfill disposal (billion pounds)	Landfill greenhouse gas emissions (metric tonnes CO2e)	Avoided emissions landfill food waste was never grown (metric tonnes CO2e)
Grains	11.1	8,460,000	11,957,833
Fruits and vegetables	42.32	32,549,000	41,853,908
Dairy	15.26	11,690,000	24,937.370
Brown's produce from Figure 9.4	27,391 pounds	9.8	20.1

Source: WARM, 2015.

of most uneaten grains, fruits, vegetables, dairy products and meat in proportions provided by the USDA. For the first time, the emissions from landfilling these foods can be calculated and then compared to food waste management alternatives, such as waste prevention, donation, or composting.

Table 9.4 lists a sample of WARM model output that compares the GHG emissions of foods that are disposed of in landfills in the proportions that the USDA estimates (WARM 2015). In this scenario, food waste was proportioned among fruits and vegetables, grains, and dairy, while excluding meats and seafood from the analysis. The results illustrate that food waste is a significant contributor to greenhouse gas emission and, hence, climate change. This example highlights the climate-change benefits from not growing food that will only be wasted. The largest greenhouse gas emission reductions occur by simply preventing waste. Also, shown are the calculated GHG emissions from the produce measured in the sample from Brown's ShopRite summarized in Figure 9.4 excluding the 3,487 pounds of produce that was donated. Landfill emissions from the remaining 27,391 pounds of produce would have been 9.8 metric tons. Had that food not been grown at all, the total avoided emissions from this monthly sample would have been 20.1 metric tons, roughly equivalent to combusting nearly 2,300 gallons of gasoline.

Education and outreach: current progress and future plans

Once the decision has been made to implement innovative programs, a next step is to design promotional and training material for constituent groups. FSSM connects and engages with many different stakeholder groups each with a wide range of participants working with the stakeholder network (Figure 9.5).

It is evident that the overall structure of FSSM takes into account a wide range of the community. Each group has its own point of entry; consequently, communication outreach, marketing, and education targets are varied. Without extensive integration among the diverse groups of individuals, FSSM would never

Improving Food System Efficiency, Releaving Hunger
Creating New Foods & Economic Development

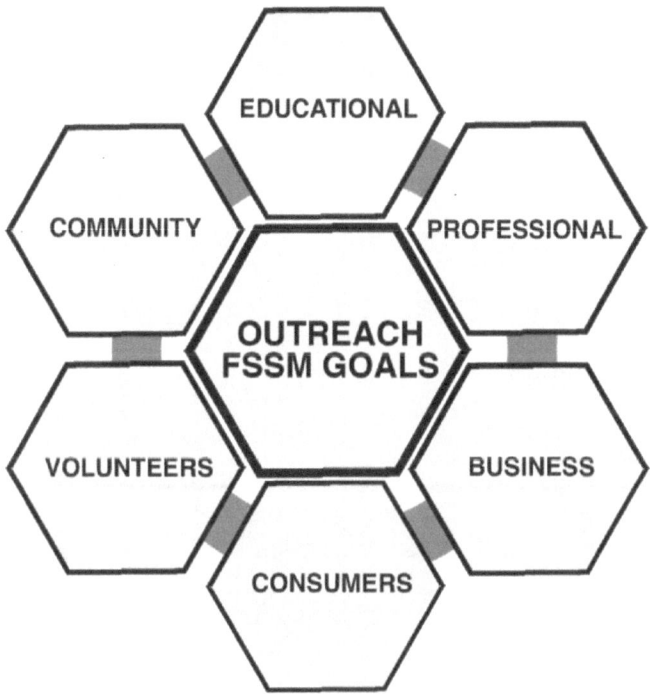

Figure 9.5 FSSM stakeholders outreach

reach its full potential for reducing food waste and contributing to economic development and healthy communities.

Communications between each of constituents groups maps onto a strategic framework of associated but unique activities, goals, and needs (Table 9.5). The business groups could be oriented towards food markets, food processors, and restaurants. Groups of supporting professionals would include marketing, environmental science, public and government relations, food scientists, public health, and chefs. Community groups, volunteers, and consumers are motivated by their provision of healthy food options and food waste reduction, which can be uniquely met by ongoing messaging. Whereas a decade ago the messages were distributed via major media outlets, current channels of communication to raise public awareness and prompt behavior change are both open and very segmented. Consequently, messages must be crafted for many media and targeted at specific audiences. Overall this analysis of the stakeholders suggests a new FSSM paradigm for dealing with food waste by engaging all of the stakeholders in new ways to communicate and explore coordinated objectives that also include improved nutrition, health, education, and economic development and job creation as key goals.

Table 9.5 Specific FSSM educational outreach, current progress, and future goals (also see Figure 9.5)

Type of participants	Activities	Goals/outcomes	Development need	Recent progress with examples
Business and professional	Food markets	Divert waste from landfills	Hunger relief and new food product development	Engaged local and national super-market chains, develop new food products and scale-up potentials
Business and professional	Food processors and large NGOs	Divert waste from landfills and give more food for hunger relief	Increase efficiency from food produce waste stream, create new products	Testing new product development from waste stream savings, develop new kitchens to scale up food savings; example, http://tinyurl.com/oc6kowr
Business and professional	Restaurants	Preventing food waste and provide training support of soup kitchen and shelter staff	New food recipes, support for community and patron's food waste reduction	Engaging local chefs and restaurants to develop new programs for surplus food, opening new restaurant for saved food
Professional educational	Training	New expertise in safety, security and sustainability	Educational Institutions need to develop classes, on line courses	New targeted on line basic courses for chefs, and for food safety practices; example, www.servingfoodsolutions.com
Consumers	Social/education experiences	Decrease in household food waste, community advocacy	Make food saving attractive, provide social media, new cost savings	Creation of new Facebook pages and means to engage food business and NGOs; example, https://www.facebook.com/WMFFoodRescue
Volunteers	Soup kitchens, shelters, NGOs	Improve acceptance, use and safety of donated foods, community advocacy	Training at local site levels, on line courses, certifications	Targeted on line courses for transferring prepared foods to shelters; example, http://communityfoodrescue.org/food-safety/safe-food-handling-videos/
Community	Increased public awareness	Support local and regional lowering of waste and better sharing of food resources	Better advertising, improved media, useful metrics, APPS, outreach to news media, social organizers	Developed public presentations and publications to local communities and also to national/international organizations; examples, The Daily News, 2014; http://www.biocycle.net/2015/10/21/food-was-never-meant-to-be-wasted

Conclusions

The sustainable potential for scalable economic, social, and environmental opportunities using FSSM is substantial. We propose that low-cost surplus foods are ideal for safely adding value for resale and reuse. Preliminary analysis suggests that local food entrepreneurs can create new business opportunities including living-wage jobs based on the advantages of successful new inputs. A market-driven approach to solving several social, economic, and environmental problems could further optimize the sustainability of the proposed FSSM outcomes.

Moving forward, numerous opportunities will depend on making the best use of available surplus produce and skill sets of a supporting team of sustainable food, culinary, education, and business specialists. Nutrition research and public health concerns are being incorporated throughout the project and FSSM approach. The Drexel Food Lab is working with local food incubators to bring test-products to the marketplace in early 2016. The Lab continues to work with Brown's Super Stores and other grocers to evaluate and test various value-added food options. Multi-media, multi-lingual educational video options with turnkey templates are planned or underway using the Targeted Open-Online Course (TOOC) format. Web-based applications are in development to improve the shift away from food waste to food saving solutions.

Drexel Food Lab, working with Brown's Super Stores, is testing how surplus produce can be profitably converted into food products using low-cost produce for manufacturing sustainable food products. In one evidenced-based simulation, we estimated surplus produce could be used for new products generating significant monthly gross revenues and net profits as well as economically feasible gross profits for local social enterprises. These scenarios illustrate the possibilities for creating profitable food businesses closely linked to the community using many different recipe and product options. Together, these data driven examples demonstrate significant cost savings and new sources of income can be immediately enacted to decrease food waste and make it available for the urban poor of the US.

FSSM is not limited to produce. The project team is now considering how to engage other foods – meat, dairy, seafood, baked goods – in the process. The methodology is also not limited to surplus foods from grocery stores. Farm fresh foods are being analyzed along with potential surplus food inputs from distributors, manufacturers, and food service bearing in mind how food products, restaurants items, and recipes for hunger relief groups are all a part of the program.

Food loss in the US is enormous. There is no lack of product to sustain FSSM, feed new social enterprises, and to prevent wastage – the willingness of new groups of people to learn how to successfully engage in FSSM is the primary and essential need.

Acknowledgements

Grateful acknowledgements are extended to the Brown's Super Store team for continuing their efforts to sustainably manage supermarkets and care for the communities they serve. Much of the research reported here is first of its kind thanks to their leadership. We also acknowledge the many students at Drexel University and Cabrini College who engaged so enthusiastically and skillfully with this project.

Disclaimer

Any views expressed in this report do not necessarily represent those of either the United States government or the Environmental Protection Agency. Mention of trade names or commercial products does not constitute endorsement or recommendation for use.

References

BAMCO, n.d., Imperfectly Delicious Produce. Available online at www.bamco.com/timeline/imperfectly-delicious-produce/ (accessed May 30, 2016).

Chokshi, N. 2014. "City Hunger and Homelessness in 10 Charts." *Washington Post*, December 12.

Church Brothers. n.d. Church Brothers to Showcase #Imperfectveg at PMA Foodservice. Available online at http://churchbrothers.com/content/?p=11688 (accessed January 18, 2016).

Daily News, Philadelphia. 2014. "Drexel Food Lab dishes up solutions for food challenges." September 9.

Eat Café. n.d. Available online at www.eatcafe.org/ (accessed May 30, 2016).

FEB. 2015. Urban Surplus Food Recovery Model Team. Available online at http://tinyurl.com/lthelsc (accessed May 30, 2016).

Feeding America. n.d. Map the Meal Gap. Available online at http://map.feedingamerica.org/county/2013/overall (accessed May 30, 2016).

FMI n.d. Supermarket Facts. Available online at www.fmi.org/research-resources/supermarket-facts (accessed May 30, 2016).

Gundersen, C., Waxman, E., Engelhard, E., Satoh, A., and Chawla, N. 2013. *Feeding America*. Chicago, Illinois

Gunders, D. 2012. "Wasted: How America Is Losing Up to 40 Percent of Its Food from Farm to Fork to Landfill." Natural Resources Defense Council, IP:12-06-B. Available online at www.nrdc.org/food/wasted-food.asp (accessed May 30, 2016).

Health.gov. n.d.. Dietary Guidelines. Available online at http://health.gov/dietaryguidelines/ (accessed May 30, 2016).

HUD Exchange. n.d. Promise Zones First Round Urban Designees. Available online at http://tinyurl.com/mju8rme (accessed May 30, 2016).

Huffington Post. 2015. Students Devise Way to Feed Homeless Meals, Cut Food Waste All at Once. Available online at www.huffingtonpost.com/2015/03/02/drexel-food-lab-homeless_n_6784098.html (accessed May 30, 2016).

Imperfect Produce. n.d. About Us. Available online at www.imperfectproduce.com/home (accessed May 30, 2016).

L.A.Kitchen. n.d. *Reclaim LA – Food Recovery*. Available online at www.lakitchen.org/reclaim-la/ (accessed May 30, 2016).

Lampert, P. 2015. *They Don't Just Cook It, They Create It*. Available online at www.supermarketguru.com/the-lempert-report/they-dont-just-cook-it,-they-create-it.html (accessed May 30, 2016).

Massachusetts. n.d. *Commercial Food Waste Disposal Ban*. Available online at http://www.mass.gov/eea/agencies/massdep/recycle/solid/massachusetts-waste-disposal-bans.html (accessed May 30, 2016).

NPR. June 17, 2015. To Tackle Food Waste, Big Grocery Chain Will Sell Produce Rejects. Available online at www.npr.org/sections/thesalt/2015/06/17/414986650/to-tackle-food-waste-big-grocery-chain-will-sell-produce-rejects (accessed May 30, 2016).

O'Donnell, T. 2014. Cobbler Cure – Doctors Orders. Available online at tinyurl.com/kxlss85 (accessed May 30, 2016).

O'Donnell, T.H., Deutsch, J., Yungmann, C., Zeitz, A. and Katz, S.H. 2015a. "New sustainable market, opportunities for surplus food: A food system-sensitive methodology (FSSM)." *Food and Nutrition Sciences* 6: 883–892. Available online at http://dx.doi.org/10.4236/fns.2015.610093 (accessed May 30, 2016).

O'Donnell, T.H., Deutsch, J., Pepino, R., Millron, B.J., Yungmann, C., and Katz, S.H. 2015b. "Food was never meant to be wasted." *Biocycle*, October, 2015, 34–38.

Robinson Fresh. n.d. To Tackle Food Waste, Big Grocery Chain Will Sell Produce Rejects. Available online at www.npr.org/sections/thesalt/2015/06/17/414986650/to-tackle-food-waste-big-grocery-chain-will-sell-produce-rejects (accessed May 30, 2016).

Schwaner-Albright, O. 2015. "Five-Star Dining on Leftover Scraps?" *Wall Street Journal*, June 12.

Seymour, G., Tucker, G.A., Poole, M. and Giovannoni, J. 2013. *The Molecular Biology and Biochemistry of Fruit Ripening*. Oxford: Wiley-Blackwell. Available online at http://dx.doi.org/10.1002/9781118593714 (accessed May 30, 2016).

SFEnvironment. n.d. *Recycling and Composting*. http://www.sfenvironment.org/zero-waste/recycling-and-composting (accessed May 30, 2016).

SFGate. March 19, 2015. To Tackle Food Waste, Big Grocery Chain Will Sell Produce Rejects. Available online at http://insidescoopsf.sfgate.com/blog/2015/03/19/imperfectly-delicious-produce-a-new-outlet-for-ugly-but-good-produce/ (accessed May 30, 2016).

Shelby Report. 2015. Associated Food Stores Offers 'Misfit' Robinson Fresh Produce. Available online at www.theshelbyreport.com/2015/10/03/associated-food-stores-offers-misfit-robinson-fresh-produce-for-halloween/ (accessed May 30, 2016).

Sustainable Development. n.d. Sustainable Development Goal 12.3. Available online at https://sustainabledevelopment.un.org/?menu=1300 (accessed May 30, 2016).

The Real Junk Food Project. n.d. *Welcome to the Real Junk Food Project*. Available online at http://therealjunkfoodproject.org/ (accessed May 30, 2016).

The U.S. Conference of Mayors. 2014. *Hunger & Homelessness, 2014*. Washington, DC: City Policy Associates, 112 p. Available online at www. usmayors.org/pressreleases/uploads/2014/1211-report-hh.pdf (accessed May 30, 2016).

USDA(a). n.d. *USDA and EPA Join with Private Sector, Charitable Organizations to Set Nation's First Food Waste Reduction Goals*. Available online at http://tinyurl.com/p2df297 (accessed May 30, 2016).

USDA(b). n.d. *Supplemental Nutrition Assistance Program*. Available online at www.fns.usda.gov/snap/supplemental-nutrition-assistance-program-snap (accessed May 30, 2016).

USDA(c). n.d. Available online at www.usda.gov/oce/foodwaste/faqs.htm (accessed May 30, 2016).

USDA(d). n.d. Food Security Status of U.S. Households in 2014. Available online at www.ers.usda.gov/topics/food-nutrition-assistance/food-security-in-the-us/key-statistics-graphics.aspx#insecure (accessed May 30, 2016).

USDA1. n.d. *Food Availability (per Capita) Data System 2010.* U.S. Department of Agriculture Economic Research Service. Available online at http://ers.usda.gov/data-products/food-availability-(per-capita)-data-system.aspx (accessed May 30, 2016).

USDA, FNS. n.d. Diet Quality of Americans by SNAP Participation Status. Available online at www.fns.usda.gov/sites/default/files/ops/NHANES-SNAP07-10.pdf (Exhibit 5, pg xi) (accessed May 30, 2016).

USEPA (a). n.d. *Sustainable Management of Food.* Available online at www2.epa.gov/sustainable-management-food (accessed May 30, 2016).

USEPA. n.d. *Waste Reduction Model documentation.* Available online at www.epa.gov/warm (accessed May 30, 2016).

USEPA(b). 2016. *U.S. Greenhouse Gas Inventory Report: 1990–2014.* Available online at https://www3.epa.gov/climatechange/ghgemissions/usinventoryreport.html (accessed May 30, 2016).

WARM. 2015. *Food Waste, Exhibit* 14. Available online at https://www3.epa.gov/epawaste/conserve/tools/warm/pdfs/Food_Waste.pdf (accessed May 30, 2016).

YouTube. 2014. Gina McCarthy speaks at our Center for Hospitality and Sport Management. Available online at www.youtube.com/watch?v=31CYcEzaIKU (accessed May 30, 2016).

Part III

Ensuring food system resilience

10 Food safety and the emergency food supply chain

Lessons from North Carolina
food pantries

Ashley Chaifetz and Benjamin Chapman

The safety of the American food supply impacts all races, ethnicities, ages, and income levels. Every year, an estimated 48 million Americans (1 in 6) contract foodborne illnesses (Scallan et al. 2011a; Scallan et al. 2011b) from grocery stores, hospitals, prisons, church banquets, county fairs, restaurants, private homes, schools, and even meal programs like Meals on Wheels (Centers for Disease Control and Prevention 2011; Vail 2015). The estimated cost of foodborne illness in America each year is $36 billion, with an average case cost of $3,630 per illness (Minor et al. 2014).

Only recently have researchers begun to examine the risk of foodborne illness for food-insecure populations, particularly when it comes to emergency foods (Henley et al. 2012; Koro et al. 2010; Quinlan 2013). "Emergency food" is the overarching term for foods distributed to food-insecure populations through shelters, food banks, food pantries, soup kitchens, backpack programs, and other institution-specific programs. Food banks and pantries are the largest part of the emergency food system. Food banks are large warehouse operations that store and distribute food from producers, retailers, federal commodity programs, and the food industry to the food pantries, which distribute emergency food at the local level (Berner and O'Brien 2004; Curtis and McClellan 1995). To further clarify, food pantries are the locations where individuals and families go to obtain food, whereas the food banks distribute to their food pantry partners. More often than not, food pantries are affiliated with or located in a church or religious organization, though one rarely needs to be affiliated to obtain food.

Unlike the supply chain that ends at the grocery store, non-profit hunger relief organizations rely largely on donations, and only some consistently know when they will receive a food donation or the details of its transport. Even with pantry participation in federal programs like The Emergency Food Assistance Program (TEFAP) and the Supplemental Nutrition Assistance Program (SNAP 2013), emergency food tends to be stationed outside the traditional market, its supply chain understudied and forgotten. TEFAP is a federal program of the United States Department of Agriculture that provides no-cost food to the states for low-income and elderly individuals and families. The states give the food to selected organizations, predominately food banks, which distribute the items to local non-profit agencies like food pantries, soup kitchens, and homeless shelters. While most SNAP benefits are in the form of food stamps for grocery store use, the program also distributes non-perishable foods to food banks and food pantries, typically alongside TEFAP.

More than one-quarter of the 9.9 million residents of North Carolina are classified as food-insecure, as measured by the prevalence of limited food per paycheck, the cost of goods, persistent feelings of hunger, and lack of money for food (Feeding America 2013; Coleman-Jensen et al. 2012). They are served by a network of food banks and food pantries, many affiliated with Feeding America, the nation's largest domestic hunger relief charity, which provides 46.5 million people with 3.3 billion meals annually via its 200 member food banks and 60,000 food pantries (Feeding America 2014). This network relies heavily on corporate sponsorship, retail and manufacturing donations, and federal commodity programs, TEFAP in particular. Feeding America and its partners distribute 80 percent of all TEFAP items in the country (Feeding America 2014). Grocery stores and food drives play a large role in emergency food redistribution (Schneider 2013), but food also comes from a variety of sources, including individual donations, community gardens, local farms, and leftovers from restaurants (Bhattarai et al. 2005; Curtis and McClellan 1995; Daponte and Bade 2006; Davis et al. 2014; Teron and Tarasuk 1999).

This variability in food sources raised concerns about emergency food safety, liability and financial responsibility for illnesses and resulted in passage of the Bill Emerson Good Samaritan Food Donation Act 1996. which alleviates liability concerns for foods donated in good faith (Morenoff 2002). The Act, which has since been applied by all states, was passed because large grocery chains were hesitant to donate expired and nearly-expired foods due to liability concerns (Cohen 2006). While the legislation reduced questions regarding the donor's incentive to take care, it does not necessarily prohibit any particular foods for donation. To use a phrase coined by Parker et al., the supply chains and operating procedures of food pantries adhere to a "loosely-coupled system of standards," meaning that there is no overarching rule that the pantries follow (Parker et al. 2012).

Beyond the dictates of the Bill Emerson Good Samaritan Act, food pantries in North Carolina must adhere North Carolina law that requires donated meat products to come from an inspected source, be free of microbiological spoilage, and kept stored under adequate refrigeration temperature (2 N.C.A.C. 9C.0304 2013). However, the pantries themselves are not inspected. Moreover, critics argue that there is a dearth of publicly available information regarding food safety for the approximately 2,500 food pantry managers in North Carolina. Without clear regulations, many food pantries create their own rules and procedures with respect to food safety, though they are rarely formalized (Chaifetz and Chapman 2015).

The emergency food system poses unique challenges to food safety. Individuals with limited resources use various strategies to feed themselves and their families—foods that can include "road kill," crops gleaned from fields, and salvaged goods (Anater et al. 2011; Kempson et al. 2002a; Kempson et al. 2002b; Kempson et al. 2003). The lack of grocery store access can lead individuals to alternative food sources, including food pantries (Blanchard and Matthews 2007; Smith and Morton 2009). Those foods, alongside foods obtained for pantry donation, can travel varying distances with varying levels of risk: hot backseats and trunks of cars, refrigerated vans, and so forth. As such, inconsistent and unregulated donated foods are thought to be of higher risk when compared to traditional retail purchased foods (Finch and Daniel 2005). Additionally and more importantly, food handlers in the emergency food system are typically volunteers. The role of the pantries and their volunteers in food provision is critical, yet excluded from food handling research.

The supply chain literature does not focus on what happens to food post-purchase – that is, when the foods move to the emergency food providers. There is an unknown level of risk regarding each product and minimizing that risk is critical for all pantries and products. While many members of the public understand that a foodborne illness outbreak is an evolving process they want the ability to make "fully informed food choices under conditions of risk uncertainty through the presentation of all relevant information in an understandable and intelligible way" (Frewer et al. 2002: 370). Managers, volunteers, and clients of food pantries may or may not have the relevant information (Chaifetz and Chapman 2015). The emergency food supply chain differs from a traditional supply chain in many ways, but most importantly, the recipients of the items (i.e., the food pantries) have little control over it.

This chapter describes and begins the empirical analysis of the supply chain of redistributed goods using a novel data set. Its purpose is to characterize the supply process and provide insight on improvement regarding food safety in the North Carolina emergency food supply chain, addressing transport practices, storage procedures, and gaps in knowledge. Supply chains are generally complex. Lambert and Cooper (2000: 65) explain, "The supply chain is not a chain of businesses with one-to-one, business-to-business relationships, but a network of multiple businesses and relationships." However, we have remarkably little understanding of the emergency food system, itself dependent on myriad supply chains, particularly when it comes to food safety. While some food sources are expected, like grocery stores and federal government commodities, the likelihood and frequency of garden harvest, hunted game, gleaned fruits and vegetables, salvaged leftover catered and restaurant meals, and even meat and dairy from local producers remains uncertain, as do the means of transport and containers. Such gaps are important especially as the clients have limited resources in the event of foodborne illness.

Methodology

With more than 2,500 food pantries in North Carolina, a stratified random sample of 12 (of 100) counties was used to achieve a generalizable and representative sample of the state that could later be extrapolated to the larger American population. Levels of food security and poverty were considered as variables for stratification, but food security rates are correlated with population in both populous and sparse counties. All counties in North Carolina that have at least 25 percent of the population in poverty have fewer than 60,000 people (USDA 2013; SNAP 2013). Given that correlation, four categories were created based on the nine urban, rural, and metropolitan divisions used by the U.S. Census Bureau. A random number generator was used to achieve 12 counties: 6 in metropolitan statistical areas, 4 in "micropolitan" areas – defined as regions with at least one area of 10,000 people but no more than 50,000 – and 2 rural counties not adjacent to metro areas.

A list of food pantries was created for the 12 counties, with relevant names, addresses, phone numbers, emails, and days/times of operation. In addition to reviewing publicly available information on the North Carolina food bank websites, Web searches were conducted for food pantries using the word "food pantry" or "pantry" alongside a variety of terms, including county names. The Executive Director of the North Carolina Association of Feeding America Food Banks introduced the researcher by email to requisite individuals at each food bank, some who then provided their partner (pantry) lists. Each of the seven food banks is responsible for a region of seven to more than 30 counties, plus partial counties. All 282 known pantries in the 12 counties were contacted, resulting in 105 interviews—a 37.2 percent response rate. The pantry managers were informed in the first conversation or email that the research focused on food safety and would require both an interview and the collection of observational pantry data. Each pantry was contacted twice, either by phone or email initially, and by phone in the second attempt. On-site visits and interviews occurred from February to June 2014. While the study is limited due to the selection bias of the participants, the estimated impact of that bias on the supply chain analysis is minimal.

A partially-structured interview was designed and executed to identify, describe, categorize, and analyze the supply chain for North Carolina food pantries. The interview, conducted as part of the companion study regarding standard operating procedures (Chaifetz and Chapman 2015), consisted of eight multi-part questions on the sources of food distributed at the pantry, the respective delivery methods, length of travel from the suppliers, regularity of sources, and percentage of all foods from each source. Other questions resulted in the description of the kinds of foods donated, storage procedure (refrigerator, freezer, pantry, no on-site storage), any supplier requirements, repackaging and processing details, and traceability of items held on-site. The questions are both open-ended and discrete (yes-no). Content validity was assessed and the questions were pilot-tested for accuracy and extensiveness on two pantry managers outside the sample counties and by North Carolina Cooperative Extension researchers. The Institutional Review Boards of the University of North Carolina at Chapel Hill and North Carolina State University reviewed the study and its components, determining it to be "non-human subjects research."

Each interview and food pantry observation lasted from 40 minutes to 2 hours, depending on the verbosity of the manager and the busyness of the pantry. Each participant consented orally to the interview. The participating pantry managers did not receive any compensation. Each interview was typed or handwritten during the conversation; interviews initially handwritten were typed at a later date. When possible, the pantry was visited during food distribution or while bags were packed (n=70); otherwise, the pantry manager explained the organization's procedures and provided a full tour of the pantry (n=35).

To address concerns about confidentiality, participants were informed that pseudonyms for the individuals and food pantries would be used in any publications, that participation is voluntary, and that questions could be skipped at any time. Interviews were conducted in a space at the food pantry chosen by the participant. Oftentimes, the participant would answer the questions at the same time as providing a tour of the pantry and its operations, though some interviews were conducted while seated. To provide an environment of trust, the intention of the interviewer was to display interest in the participant, avoid reactionary responses, and be mindful of time.

Each interview was manually coded by assigning a unique identifier to each pantry. The variables and codes were entered into an Excel spreadsheet to count, summarize, and categorize trends in participant responses; then, the data were entered into STATA 11.2 for quantitative analysis. Data are considered statistically significant at the 90 percent confidence level (p<0.10). No missing data were imputed. Mean scores and standard deviations were calculated for each question. Two-sample t-tests were performed on various pantry characteristics, including distance from supplier, traceability, and on-site storage facilities. Passages from the full interviews were also coded in NVivo 10, allowing for analysis based on certain themes. The qualitative analysis provides reasoning behind certain actions and operating procedures.

Results

Distribution and storage

Of the pantries that participated (n=105), 83.8 percent are partnered with at least one food bank. Three food pantries are entirely mobile; no food is stored, but is distributed directly from the food bank's vehicle. Given disparities across counties and food bank regions, the pantries are not equally distributed across food bank regions, with only 23.3 percent associated with a single food bank. Most food pantries in the sample (78.1 percent) distribute both perishable and non-perishable items, with an additional 11.4 percent serving food prepared in an on-site kitchen as well as distributing bags of food. Few pantries (8.6 percent) distribute only non-perishable foods. Of the pantries that partner with a food bank (n=88), 70.5 percent participate in at least one federal commodity program, either TEFAP or SNAP or both. Both TEFAP and SNAP items are available to approved pantries depending on availability, administrative upkeep, and storage facilities. While TEFAP provides predominately non-perishable food to the food banks, it also includes fresh and frozen fruit and meat products (TEFAP 2013). A participating organization must be able to take any items provided through the program, which requires a freezer for participation. As a rule, the TEFAP and SNAP items must be stored on separate shelves than other pantry items, although interpretations of this rule tend to vary.

The majority (97.1 percent) of all visited pantries have an on-site pantry or closet for storing items, the remaining are the mobile markets. Most (80.9 percent) pantry managers have access to a refrigerator or walk-in cooler to store perishable items, while even more (88.6 percent) have access to a chest freezer, upright freezer, or walk-in freezer for storage. This said, access to cold storage does not mean that the space is unlimited. In terms of frequency of items distributed, 48.6 percent of the pantries distribute fresh dairy products (shelf-stable milk is considered a packaged item), 43.8 percent distribute eggs, 88.6 percent distribute fruits and vegetables, 85.7 percent distribute meat (which includes chicken, pork, and beef), 63.8 percent distribute deli meat, 16.2 percent distribute home-canned or processed goods, 12.4 percent distribute hunted game, and 20 percent distribute leftovers from restaurants and catered events. We did not seek specificities as to how each of those kinds of items travels to the pantries.

Storage options are limited: the volunteers distribute the items immediately, store in a refrigerator or freezer (sometimes a walk-in model), or put onto the shelves in the pantry itself. Canned and packaged items are always stored on pantry shelves. The highest risk items are the perishable items that are not stored in a cold environment. To illustrate, 93 pantries distribute fruits and vegetables and 28.0 percent of them store those items in the pantry. No pantry managers indicated that they store meat in the pantry, but some leave meat on the counter throughout the hours of distribution and others do the same with dairy products and eggs. While this action might seem innocuous, such perishable items require cold storage to better guarantee safety.

Food sources

On average, a single pantry receives food from 3.73 sources, with a minimum of one and a maximum of 16 source categories. For the food pantries that have a partnership with a food bank, it tends to be the largest source of food (71.5 percent); however, only 14 pantry managers interviewed receive 100 percent of the food from their food bank partner. Each pantry manager also explained approximately how much food was received from each category, with the average amounts listed in Table 10.1. While food banks and food drives continue to be the most common sources of food, a quarter of all pantries use grocery stores, discount grocery stores, and/or local farms and gardens (community, school, and prison) as additional sources.

Even though many food pantries distribute home-processed foods, it makes up a very small percentage of the total food distributed from that pantry (0.7 percent). Yet, the risk of contamination is higher for the home-processed canned items, given the uncertainty of their processing procedures. As a result, acceptance and distribution of home-processed foods is discouraged across all food bank regions, but the advice is inconsistently followed in both metropolitan and micropolitan areas; almost one in five managers distribute (or allow for the distribution of)

Table 10.1 Sources of food

Food source	No. of pantries using source	Average % of food from source by volume
Food bank	87	71.5%
Restaurants	24	5.5%
Grocery stores	51	24.1%
Big box stores	24	12.4%
Discount grocery stores	27	21.2%
Salvage grocery stores	2	2.5%
Home-processed	17	0.7%
Local farms	30	4.4%
Gardens	33	6.1%
Food drives	75	21.3%
Hunted game	13	2.9%
Other sources	7	38.0%

Note: The "other" category is a food source not otherwise indicated, typically a distributor or local food corporation.

home-processed items. One of the pantries canned food on-site and an inquiry into methodology resulted in the response, "these are not recipe foods." Additionally, food pantry staff often places home-canned items on a shelf designated as "take at your own risk," a system designed to encourage clients to take hard-to-distribute foods, like those that are past-date – which are not inherently unsafe. Often coupled with low-risk items, the food pantry clients are not provided with the information to make an informed decision regarding the riskier home-processed foods.

With certainty, clients in metropolitan areas are likelier to receive a more diverse set of foods in the bags obtained at the food pantries – that is, the foods are likelier to come from more than one supplier. The increased number of suppliers means there is a probability of increased risk due to the multiple changes in environment (e.g., temperature, packaging, storage facility). Pantry managers indicated that they would not accept perishable items if they cannot be appropriately stored on-site or distributed immediately. Many of the managers do not know when they will receive a food donation and do not always have appropriate storage for surprise items. Donors often leave food on the doorstep of the pantry for the manager to find the next day, a critical problem due to the lack of time-temperature control.

Transportation

Unlike other food supply chains, the transportation of emergency food does not consist of one specific item, like meat, that has particular storage needs. Multiple items are transported all at once; a car trunk or even a cooler could contain dairy, meat, bread, and fruit; the vehicles are not necessarily temperature-controlled, allowing for an increased risk of contamination. Each pantry manager seeks to find food sources to fulfill its client base and does so as needed—with one source or up to ten sources. Figure 10.1 summarizes the overall supply chain options for any single food pantry. The product flow, or supply chain, for food pantry items is especially difficult to chart, given its complex nature.

Food from the food bank also comes from numerous sources, each which traveled varying lengths of time and in unknown conditions to arrive at the food bank, where it remains until a food pantry manager retrieves it. Meat is an especially popular item among clients, characterized by managerial sentiments "the more meat, the more people" and "people will wait in a line for meat." For a product as simple as hunted venison, an individual could process it at home or give it to a certified processor via an organization like Hunters for the Hungry or

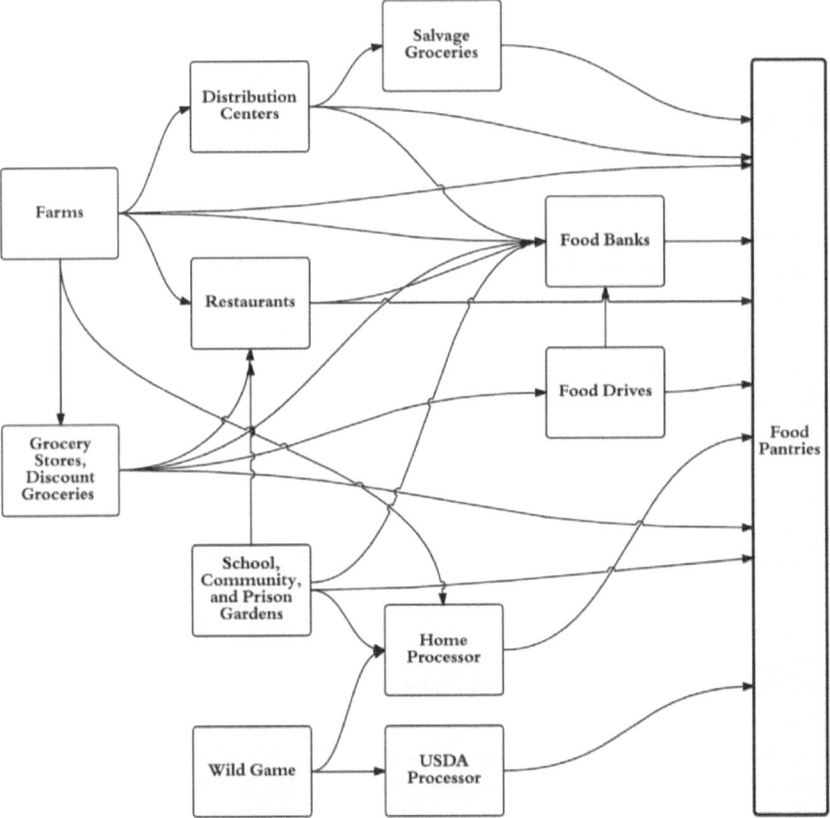

Figure 10.1 Supply chain for food pantries

Notes: This figure does not include the supply chain for the items directly before they arrive at grocery stores, restaurants, or distribution centers, only the sources directly before the pantry. The parts of this supply chain that are entirely unregulated include: school, community, and prison gardens, wild game, any home-processed items (including game), and the food pantries.

Backyard Bow Pro, both prominent in parts of North Carolina. A single food pantry tends to receive a single type of product (e.g., meat) from numerous sources, multiple times per week. For example, eggs can be purchased in a store, delivered from a farm, or even come from one's personal henhouse. Only one pantry in the sample candled eggs on-site to check on the growth of the embryo, a sign that the egg has been fertilized. The food pantry managers and volunteers use their discretion to decide whether the product is safe or "good enough" to distribute.

Of the pantries that get vegetables from community, school, and even prison gardens, 21.2 percent have a garden on site. Of the 30 pantries that receive produce (sometimes gleaned) from farms, 83.3 percent of them have those items delivered, sometimes by the farmers themselves. Gardens and farms have their own operating procedures that may or may not follow best practices, leading to variable foodborne illness risk.

Methods of delivery

Many food donors offer a mixture of both non-perishable and perishable goods, some frozen and some refrigerated, both requiring low temperatures so that the items do not defrost or get into the "danger zone" above 41°F (United States Department of Health and Human Services 2009). However, outside the food bank, a refrigerated truck is not a common method of transport. Most pantry managers pick up food bank items in a personal vehicle, be it car, truck, or organizational van. While some pantry managers explained that they used coolers for transport (typically required by the large grocery chains to pick up food), few stated that they used freezer blankets. For the most part, a pick-up from the food bank often requires more space than a typical sedan, leading to the rental or borrowing of trailers, box trucks, vans, and pick-up trucks, especially if the items include TEFAP or SNAP commodities, which tend to be in bulk. Few other donations are similar in size or require special transportation.

Transport times

Used as a regulatory framework in North Carolina, the 2009 Model Food Code stipulates that four hours is the maximum length of time that food can be left without refrigeration before it must be discarded (United States Department of Health and Human Services 2009). Because mileage by itself fails to capture the length of time for potential temperature shifts while food is in transit, we instead use the average number of minutes the food travels from one point to another from each type of food source, as shown in Table 10.2. Of note, the food from the food banks dwarfs any other source in terms of maximum time to destination, and 46.7 percent pantry managers explained that it takes more than 30 minutes for the food to travel to the pantry. Another 10.5 percent stated it took at least one hour, and as many as two hours. While the actual length of time in transit may be understated if food is delivered by truck from a distant food bank (or any other source) and the truck makes multiple stops, all pantries indicated the time in transit was fewer

Table 10.2 Food transit times (N=105)

Food source	Average no. of minutes in transit	Median transit time	Min. transit time	Max. transit time	% of pantries that could not report transit times[+]
Food bank	46.4	45	5	120	20.7%
Restaurants	14.7	11	2	45	45.8%
Grocery stores	10.1	6.5	1	90	29.4%
Big box stores	19.1	15	2	90	25.0%
Discount grocery stores	14.1	10	2	75	25.9%
Salvage grocery stores	7	7	7	7	50.0%
Home-processed	4	5	1	5	76.5%
Local farms	7.8	8	5	10	86.7%
Gardens	1.1	1	1	2	76.5%
Food drives	8.6	4	1	30	82.3%
Hunted game	5	5	5	5	92.3%
Other sources	11	11	2	20	71.4%

Note: All times in minutes.
[+]This percentage is only of the food pantries that distribute said items, not of all pantries.

than four hours. Two-sample t-tests were performed on the distances from each location type to understand any statistically significant differences between the pantries that did and did not partner with a food bank. The sample in this analysis only includes the food pantries that used said source for each question.

The distances from the grocery stores ($p<0.05$) and farms ($p<0.05$) were each associated with statistically significant differences in food bank partnership even with small sample sizes (n=36 and n=4, respectively). For the other locations, there was no statistically significant difference between the pantries that do and do not partner with a food bank. Correspondingly, two-sample t-tests were also performed on the distances from each location type to determine any statistically significant differences between the pantries that are and are not in metropolitan areas. This analysis should be more robust, given that the pantries in metropolitan areas are likelier to have access to numerous sources, but these results only somewhat validate earlier hypotheses regarding food access. The average time in transit is lengthier when the pantry is in a non-metropolitan area, but not statistically different. The food pantries that distribute hunted game rarely knew from how far it came.

The lack of knowledge by pantry managers as to how long and far food travels before delivery (Table 10.2) is critical due to the potential lack of temperature control. Anecdotally, perishable items sometimes remain in car trunks or truck beds before they arrive at the pantry. Food drive items tend to be packaged or canned, the time in transit matters less than if the food is highly perishable. In the case of food drives, individuals typically deliver the food to the church or organization and the pantry manager retrieves it from a bin on site.

Traceability

Traceability is the ease by which the manager would be able to determine the original source of an item. This question was asked to determine how difficult it would be to react to an ill client claiming foodborne illness contraction from an item in the pantry. To further explain, during the interview, items from six categories were chosen for questioning: grain, meat, packaged (can, package, or jar) items, fruits and vegetables, eggs, and dairy. The interviewer asked about the item's origin (supplier) and length of time spent in the pantry. Most pantry managers were able to trace the items in question, even though products like fruits and vegetables do not have labels and often get combined with other like items. Conversely, packaged goods were the hardest to trace, but they are clearly labeled by brand. Once packaged items are categorized within the pantry (for example, all cans of corn together, regardless of brand), they are harder to trace based on supplier. Given that TEFAP and SNAP items have identifying (non-brand) labels, certain food bank items tended to be simpler to trace. None of the home-processed foods were labeled with details on how the food was processed, with few labeled at all. Without labels, it would be difficult to find the contamination source in the event of foodborne illness.

Given the sheer number of food pantries that are partnered with a food bank, it would seem as though a few independent pantries could skew the analysis. Two-sample t-tests on the pantry manager's ability to trace the sources of certain items were performed to test any statistically significant differences between them. For pantries that distribute fruits and vegetables and are partnered with a food bank, those managers are better able to trace the source of the product, statistically significant at the 95 percent confidence level. The distribution of other items revealed no statistically significant differences based on food bank partnership, meaning that the food bank partnership bears little influence on traceability.

Even with the small sample size, the pantries were further divided into groups: food bank partners in metropolitan and non-metropolitan areas. The pantries in rural areas did not reveal the statistically significant differences initially hypothesized, at least in terms of traceability of their food items. Here, the food pantries not located in metropolitan areas were better able to trace their canned goods, statistically significant at the 95 percent confidence level. A divide in food access may remain, but the within-pantry differences based on population are lacking. Overall, canned goods have less risk for contamination on site, as they do not require freezing or refrigeration. Given the package labels, they are generally easier to trace than fruits and vegetables.

Limitations of this research

While the overall supply chain (Figure 10.1) might be generalizable to food pantry supply chains nationwide, this analysis allows for continued uncertainty on delivery mechanisms and sources in other states, as state regulations and food bank rules differ from North Carolina. Metropolitan areas in North Carolina might not mirror those of much-larger metropolitan areas, like New York, Los Angeles, or Houston. Larger networks and accessibility to foods of all kinds might allow for increased diversity of sources and foods. However, the impact of poor practices varies amongst pantries, as some pantries distribute to ten families per month and others to hundreds.

While this sample is purposeful, threats to internal validity could be reduced with a larger sample of food pantries. Managers who were discouraged by the inclusion of the food safety language in the email might also be those who are least confident in their practices, meaning that the analysis in this paper is the upper bound. To that end, the pantries that are "riskier" are likely to be doing more activities within the pantries, from transporting and storing more types of items to receiving food from myriad locations. The pantries that only distribute non-perishables or only have foods from the food bank have fewer potential ways to increase or decrease their respective scores.

Conclusions and future research

The food pantries in North Carolina and across the country depend on philanthropic endeavors from grocery stores, farms and individuals. Given the lack of regulation and formal recommendations to foods pantries in North Carolina, personal beliefs regarding food safety prevail at the pantry-level. While food banks have refrigerators and freezers, as well as dedicated staff and food safety policies, the supply chain is intrinsically complicated to understand. The food pantries lack formal contingency plans and fail to evaluate their suppliers for any sort of supply risk. The dearth of professional staff might play a role, though the literature has not yet evaluated that aspect. If a risk has not yet materialized into known foodborne illness, it might be difficult to justify any time and cost of its mitigation, as the lack of illness suggests the lack of a problem. There are likely many points along the supply chain that are risky, rather than one centralized problem, and outside factors might be correlated with those risky choices.

While this analysis adds to the literature, it remains incomplete. A comparative case study of high-risk items and their specific supply chains would allow for a richness not provided. It is unlikely that the pantries will invest in refrigerated trucks given the expense, but increased information on and access to coolers and freezer blankets would lessen risks of microbial growth due to a lack of time-temperature control. As for the increased distribution of perishable items like dairy, fruits and vegetables, and meat, pantry managers would be able to accept a full pallet of a particular item if they had the space for its contents, or if there was a way to share with other emergency food distributors in the area, including but not limited to soup kitchens and shelters.

From a policy perspective, this chapter provides support for certain operating procedures over others (e.g., storage facilities) and dispels the notion that the rurally located food pantries operate in significantly different way than those in metropolitan areas. Limited regulatory policy regarding time-temperature control and proper storage could improve supply chain procedures, as would providing educational materials, so that managers and volunteers would have full information regarding foodborne illness risk. Food banks might also be an ideal institution to support, implement, and enforce such policies for their partners. They might also be able to assist with increasing cold storage on-site so that the pantries are capable of accepting more perishable items. Food pantry managers should learn more about the mechanisms that drive the supply chain – from how the food is delivered to the length of time it spends in the car's trunk. To that end, the pantry managers can supply their volunteers with instructional information and details on the best ways to transport food and keep it as safe as possible.

Millions of people in North Carolina and across the country depend on the emergency food system. Given that system's complexity, it is necessary for policymakers and researchers alike to better understand that system and work to ensure its greater safety. From a normative perspective, all people should have access to the safest food possible – not just those who have the money to pay for it. It is a public health failure if individuals who obtain emergency food get sick from consuming it. Current and future research can add to the richness of this field by incorporating details on the emergency food supply chain and food acquisition practices centered on food-insecure populations, stagnant at almost one in seven Americans (Coleman-Jensen et al. 2012). The research regarding the United States emergency food system remains incomplete.

Acknowledgements

This project was also supported, in part, by Agriculture and Food Research Initiative Competitive grant 2012-68003-30155 from the U.S. Department of Agriculture, National Institute of Food and Agriculture and a Leland J. Bellòt Summer Research Fellowship from the Graduate School of the University of North Carolina at Chapel Hill.

References

2 N.C.A.C. 9C.0304. 2013. *Reconditioning and labeling*. Available online at http://reports. oah.state.nc.us/ncac/title%2002%20-%20agriculture%20and%20consumer%20 services/chapter%2009%20-%20food%20and%20drug%20protection/subchapter%20 c/02%20ncac%2009c%20.0304.doc (accessed February 14, 2014).

Anater, A., McWilliams, R., and Latkin, C. 2011. Food acquisition practices used by food-insecure individuals when they are concerned about having sufficient food for themselves and their households. *Journal of Hunger and Environmental Nutrition*, 6(1): 27–44.

Berner, M., and O'Brien, K. 2004. The shifting pattern of food security support: Food stamp and food bank usage in North Carolina. *Nonprofit and Voluntary Sector Quarterly*, 33(4): 655–672.

Bhattarai, G.R., Duffy, P.A., and Raymond, J. 2005. Use of food pantries and food stamps in low-income households in the United States. *Journal of Consumer Affairs*, 39(2): 276–298.

Blanchard, T.C., and Matthews, T.L. 2007. Retail concentration, food desserts, and food-disadvantaged communities in rural America. In C.C. Hinrichs and T.A. Lyson (Eds.), *Remarking the North American Food System: Strategies for Sustainability*. Lincoln: University of Nebraska Press.

Centers for Disease Control and Prevention. 2011. Foodborne Outbreak Online Database. Available online at wwwn.cdc.gov/foodborneoutbreaks/ (accessed December 6, 2013).

Chaifetz, A. and Chapman, B. 2015. Evaluating North Carolina food pantry food safety-related operating procedures. *Journal of Food Protection*, 78(11): 2033–2042.

Cohen, J.A. 2006. Ten years of leftovers with many hungry still left over: A decade of donations under the Bill Emerson Good Samaritan Food Donation Act. *Seattle Journal for Social Justice*, 5(1): 455–496.

Coleman-Jensen, A., Nord, M., and Singh, A. 2013. *Household food security in the United States in 2012*. USDA Economic Research Service. Report Number 155. Available online at www.ers.usda.gov/ersDownloadHandler.ashx?file=/media/1183208/err-155.pdf (accessed December 6, 2013).

Curtis, K.A., and McClellan, S. 1995. Falling through the safety net: Poverty, food assistance, and shopping constraints in an American city. *Urban Anthropology*, 24(1–2): 93–135.

Daponte, B., and Bade, S. 2006. How the private food assistance network evolved: Interactions between public and private responses to hunger. *Nonprofit and Voluntary Sector Quarterly*, 35(4): 668–690.

Davis, L.B., Sengyl, I., Ivy, J.S., Brock, III, L.G., and Miles, L. 2014. Scheduling food bank collections and deliveries to ensure food safety and improve access. *Socio-Economic Planning Sciences*, 48(3): 175–188.

Feeding America. 2013. *Map the Meal Gap*. Available online at http://feedingamerica.org/hunger-in-america/hunger-studies/map-the-meal-gap.aspx (accessed December 6, 2013).

Feeding America. 2014. *2014 Annual Report*. Available online at www.feedingamerica.org/our-response/about-us/annual-report/2014-annual-report.pdf (accessed February 20, 2015).

Finch, C., and Daniel, E. 2005. Food safety knowledge and behavior of emergency food relief organization workers: Effects of food safety training intervention. *Journal of Environmental Health*, 67(9): 30–34.

Frewer, L.J., Miles, S., Brennan, M., Kuznesof, S., Ness, M., and Ritson, C. 2002. Public preferences for informed choice under conditions of risk uncertainty. *Public Understanding of Science*, 11(4): 363–372.

Henley, S.C., Stein, S.E., and Quinlan, J.J. 2012. Identification of unique food handling practices that could represent food safety risks for minority consumers. *Journal of Food Protection*, 75(11): 2050–2054.

Kempson, K.M., Palmer, K.D., Sadani, P.S., Ridlen, S., and Scotto, R.N. 2002a. Food management practices used by people with limited resources to maintain food sufficiency as reported by nutrition educators. *Journal of the American Dietetic Association*, 102(12): 1795–9179.

Kempson, K.M. Keenan, D.P., Sadani, P.S., and Adler, A. 2002b. Educators' reports of food acquisition practices used by limited-resource individuals to maintain food sufficiency. *Family Economics and Nutrition Review*, 14(2): 44–55.

Kempson, K.M. Keenan, D.P., Sadani, P.S., and Adler, A. 2003. Maintaining food sufficiency: Coping strategies identified by limited-resource individuals versus nutrition educators. *Journal of Nutrition Education and Behavior*, 35(4): 179–188.

Koro, M.E., Anandan, S., and Quinlan, J.J. 2010. Microbial quality of food available to populations of differing socioeconomic status. *American Journal of Preventive Medicine*, 38(5): 478–481.

Lambert, D.M., and Cooper, M.C. 2000. Issues in supply chain management. *Industrial Marketing Management*, 29(1): 65–83.

Minor, T., Lasher, A., Klontz, K., Brown, B., Nardinelli, C., and Zorn, D. 2014. The per case and total annual costs of foodborne illness in the United States. *Risk Analysis*. DOI: 10.1111/risa.12316. Available online at http://onlinelibrary.wiley.com.libproxy.lib. unc.edu/doi/10.1111/risa.12316/full (accessed February 15, 2015).

Morenoff, D.L. 2002. Lost food and liability: The Good Samaritan food donation law story. *Food and Drug LJ*, 57: 107–132.

Parker, J.S., Wilson, R.S., LeJeune, J.T., Rivers, L., and Doohan, D. 2012. An expert guide to understanding grower decisions related to fresh fruit and vegetable contamination prevention and control. *Food Control*, 26(1): 107–116.

Powell, L.M., Slater, S., Mirtcheva, D., Bao, Y., and Chaloupka, F.J. 2007. Food store availability and neighborhood characteristics in the United States. *Preventive Medicine*, 44(3): 189–195.

Quinlan, J. 2013. Foodborne illness incidence rates and food safety risks for populations of low socioeconomic status and minority race/ethnicity: A review of the literature. *International Journal of Environmental Research and Public Health*, 10(8): 3634–3652.

Scallan, E., Griffin P.M., Angulo F.J., Tauxe R.V., and Hoekstra R.M. 2011a. Foodborne illness acquired in the United States: Unspecified agents. *Emerging Infectious Diseases* [serial on the Internet]. Available online at http://dx.doi.org.libproxy.lib.unc. edu/10.3201/eid1701.P21101 (accessed March 24, 2012).

Scallan, E.M., Hoekstra, R.M., Angulo, F.J., Tauxe, R.V., Widdowson, M.-A., Roy, S.L., Jones, J.L., and Griffin, P. 2011b. Foodborne illness acquired in the United States: Major pathogens. *Emerging Infectious Diseases*, 17(1): 7–15.

Schneider, F. 2013. The evolution of food donation with respect to waste prevention. *Waste Management* 33(3): 755–63.

Selfa, T., and Qazi, J. 2005. Place, taste, or face-to-face?: Understanding producer-consumer networks in "local" food systems in Washington State. *Agriculture and Human Values*, 22(4): 451–464.

Smith, C., and Morton, L.W. 2009. Rural food deserts: Low-income perspectives on food access in Minnesota and Iowa. *Journal of Nutrition Education and Behavior*, 41(3): 176–187.

Supplemental Nutrition Assistance Program. 2013. SNAP Policy Database. US Department of Agriculture. Food and Nutrition Service. Available online at www.ers.usda.gov/ datafiles/SNAPPolicyDatabase/SNAP_Policy_Database.xlsx (accessed December 10, 2013).

Teron, A.C., and Tarasuk, V.S. 1999. Charitable food assistance: What are food bank users receiving? *Canadian Journal of Public Health*, 90(6): 382–394.

The Emergency Food Assistance Program. 2013. Food and nutrition service nutrition program fact sheet. Available online at www.fns.usda.gov/sites/default/files/pfs-tefap. pdf (accessed December 27, 2013).

United States Department of Agriculture (USDA). 2013. 2013 Rural-Urban Continuum Codes. [Data File]. Available online at www.ers.usda.gov/data-products/rural-urban-continuum-codes.aspx#.UrMngmRDt6h (accessed May 25, 2016).

United States Department of Health and Human Services. 2009. Food code. Available online at www.fda.gov/downloads/Food/GuidanceRegulation/UCM189448.pdf (accessed February 15, 2015).

Vail, J. 2015. One death linked to Norovirus outbreak. *The Chanute Tribune*. Available online at www.chanute.com/news/article_2f6f3c58-9b9b-11e4-a8bf-fbaad00300ed.html (accessed February 20, 2015).

11 Creating a resilience assessment framework for urban food systems

Kimberly Zeuli and Austin Nijhuis

Over the past decade, many city leaders in the U.S. have begun to prioritize resilience planning and disaster recovery in response to the threat of climate change and an increase in the frequency and severity of natural disasters (U.S. Department of State 2014; Weir et al. 2012; Green 2012). While New Orleans post-Katrina is the most familiar example, cities such as New York City, Norfolk, Virginia, and San Francisco also have heavily invested in resilience efforts. The Rockefeller Foundation is helping to move the resilience agenda forward through its 100 Resilient Cities initiative, launched in 2013. Although this initiative is global, it has selected 15 U.S. cities thus far.[1]

The term "resilience" in the context of climate adaptation is often used in a broad or descriptive sense. While many definitions for resilience exist, at the core are three basic principles: the ability to adapt to changing conditions, withstand disruptions, and return to pre-existing conditions. A resilient system is characterized by several key components, including flexibility, diversity, redundancy, and adaptability. Resilience planning is concerned with the time period between the immediate aftermath of a shock and the return to pre-existing conditions, rather than the short-term emergency response period (Figure 11.1).

Although the resilience of U.S. food production to climate change is being addressed nationally (Hatfield et al. 2014; Malcolm et al. 2012; Walthall et al. 2012), the capacity of urban food systems to withstand and recover from a natural disaster is not considered in most metropolitan resilience planning. Yet, food systems in metro areas disrupted by disasters may not quickly return to normal operations, potentially causing significant food access issues. For example, news sources report that New York City typically only has two to three days of food on hand during normal consumption levels (Bennet 2012; Mahanta 2013). An analysis of Toronto's energy stock estimates that residential kitchens may have a three-day supply of food, while full-scale grocery stores may have up to 17 days (Bristow and Kennedy 2013). The growth of local food manufacturing and urban agriculture also raises questions about how best to mitigate risks associated with climate change impacts at national, regional and local levels.

We propose a framework to allow cities to analyze the resilience of their food systems to specific shocks and stresses, identify critical areas of weakness, and design actions and programs to improve resilience. The framework is grounded

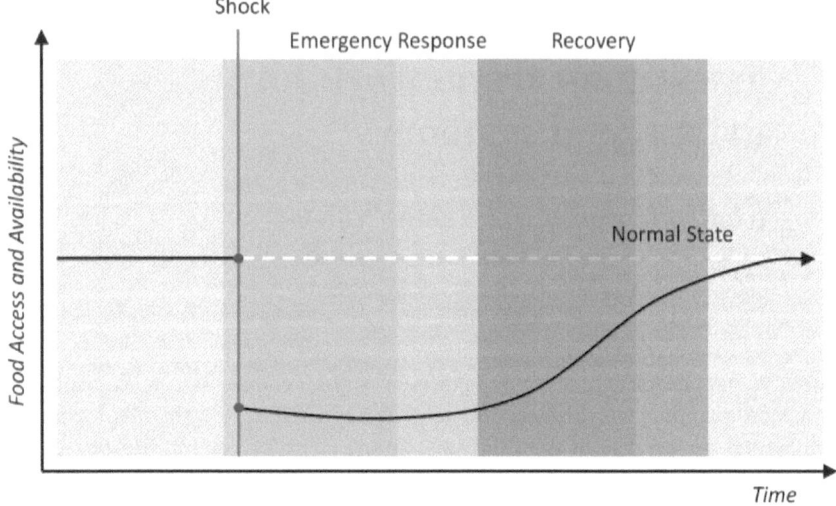

Figure 11.1 Resilience timeline
Source: Adapted from Initiative for a Competitive Inner City (2015, fig. 1).

in a thorough understanding of food system dynamics and urban food markets in the U.S. The framework and vulnerability hypotheses are discussed in the following two sections. We tested the framework in an analysis of Boston's food system in 2014–2015 and highlight the lessons learned from that study. While the strategies and actions related to Boston's food system vulnerabilities may be unique to that city, our findings support our argument that food systems should be a priority in urban resilience planning and identify key vulnerabilities that all cities should consider.

Towards a resilient food system framework

A food system comprises the three main components involved with moving and transforming food from the farm to table. Food *production* refers to all activities associated with growing crops and raising livestock. Food *processing* covers all aspects of the transformation of the food from point of production to *distribution* and includes cleaning, packaging, and processing at manufacturing facilities. For example, fresh produce such as lettuce is minimally processed, cleaned, sorted and sometimes packaged before it reaches retail outlets or restaurants. Food processed into non-perishable items, such as soup, involve more intensive manufacturing.

The distribution of food in the U.S. is a complex process that involves numerous private parties. As a result, cities do not have a clear picture of the process and all of the entities involved. There are three points along the distribution process (Figure 11.2):

1 *Packaging and manufacturing facilities*: As noted, most food stops first at a facility that sorts, packages or processes the food into a product that is sold or distributed to consumers. They are shipped in large quantities (pallets). Some produce may be shipped from the point of production directly to a mixing center or a warehouse or aggregation point.

2 *Mixing centers*: Mixing centers were created to increase supply chain efficiencies. Most retail outlets do not want a full pallet of an individual food product. Mixing centers receive pallets of individual products that are divided and combined into new pallets of multiple products for distribution centers or warehouses. Mixing centers are operated both by independent third parties and retailers that manage vertically integrated distribution systems (e.g., Walmart).

3 *Distribution centers*: Distribution centers (also called warehouses) are typically the last stop for food products before reaching a store's shelves. Large regional and national retails stores typically, but not always, own their own distribution centers. There are also regional and national distributors that manage their own centers and then distribute product to regional and local retail chains. There is also a wide range of more local distributors, many specializing in perishable food. Many cities have a large fresh food distribution center (also called a market) that serves both large grocery stores and corner stores (e.g., Hunts Point Distribution Center in New York and the San Francisco Wholesale Produce Market).

While some retail stores have vertically integrated distribution, most retail outlets, even large chains, rely on a mix of different entities to perform these various roles. As a result, and because of different food handling requirements, food products follow different paths to their shelves. For highly perishable, refrigerated products, the "cold chain" must be maintained at every point to keep the food below a specific temperature to avoid spoilage. Some food products experience a sequence of handoffs as they are shipped from production, to processing facilities, to warehouses and finally to retail outlets. Others, such as fresh produce, may have more straightforward connections between production points to retail. For some food, such as milk, producers use direct store delivery, bypassing retailer or third-party distribution centers to ship milk directly from the processing facility to retail outlets (Otto, Schoppengerd, and Shariantmadari 2009). Regardless of the distribution path, food is distributed within urban markets by trucks.

Building from the dynamics of the food system and existing body of literature, we developed a food system resilience framework that can be applied to U.S. cities. Food system resilience analysis to date has largely focused on international development settings, where food systems exhibit some fundamentally different characteristics (Fan et al. 2014; Tyler et al. 2013). Our framework was informed especially by the International Institute for Sustainable Development (IISD) and partners to analyze the resilience of food systems in Central America (Tyler et al. 2013). This said, our framework is concerned with only two parts of the food system – processing and distribution. While food production creates its own set of

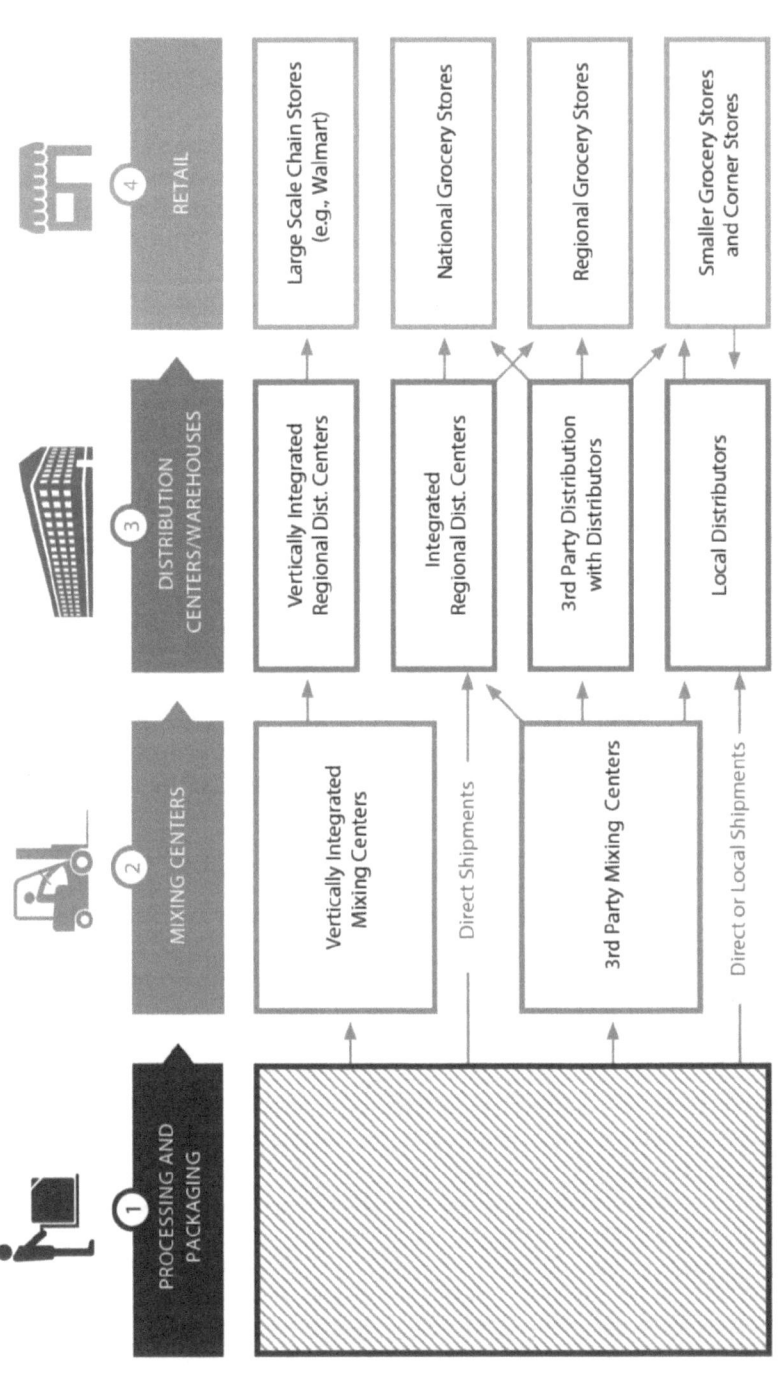

Figure 11.2 Food distribution process
Source: Adapted from Initiative for a Competitive Inner City (2015, fig. 2).

vulnerabilities (e.g., produce grown in California is at risk from drought), it is most effectively addressed at the national and international levels. Our framework was developed as a tool for city leaders to address vulnerabilities that they ostensibly can control or influence. However, the fact that the amount and origin of food supplying our cities is not known creates vulnerability. Without such data, effective planning for potential disruptions due to natural disasters or climate change is difficult.

The framework analyzes urban food systems along four components: processing and packaging; transportation and distribution; retail outlets; and food safety net (Table 11.1). These components cover the food system from the point of processing and packaging to consumer access, including purchasing food at retail locations or receiving food from food pantries and meal programs.

Potential vulnerabilities in urban food systems

The framework allows us to develop hypotheses about potential vulnerabilities within urban food systems based on economic and resilience theory (Table 11.1).

Table 11.1 Food resilience framework

Food system components	Description	Potential drivers of vulnerability
Processing and packaging	Facilities that transform food into products sold or distributed to consumers	• Concentration of facilities spatially • Concentration of companies in terms of ownership • Location of facilities in "at risk" areas • Processing and packaging regulations
Transportation and distribution	Pathways (transportation routes, facility nodes) that food products travel from processing or packaging to distribution centers and on to final point of consumer access (e.g., grocery store, food pantry, or restaurant)	• Vulnerable transportation infrastructure (e.g., weak bridges and roads, insufficient capacity, location in "at risk" areas) • Reliance on a single mode of transportation and single pathways • Vulnerabilities associated with transportation method (e.g., vehicle supply/quality, gas supply) • Lack of contingency delivery routes • Concentration of distribution facilities spatially • Concentration of distribution companies in terms of ownership • Location of distribution facilities in "at risk" areas • Distribution facilities with weak structural integrity • Distribution facilities with insufficient capacity • Sub-system distribution vulnerabilities (e.g., utilities, insufficient insurance) • Transportation and distribution regulations

Table 11.1 Continued

Food system components	Description	Potential drivers of vulnerability
Retail outlets	Outlets where consumers purchase food products (e.g., grocery stores, corner stores, bodegas, restaurants, institutions)	• Concentration of retail outlets by ownership • Location of retail outlets in "at risk" areas • Outlets have insufficient capacity, including storage to meet local demand • Outlets do not have contingency plans, including alternative supply chains and sufficient insurance • Sub-system retail outlet vulnerabilities (e.g., utilities, telecommunications for payments) • Distance to retail outlets/food deserts (sufficient retail outlets within 1-mile radius of consumers) • Vulnerabilities associated with transporting consumers to retail outlets (e.g., infrastructure, public transportation) • Ability of consumers to afford to purchase food • Retail regulations
Food safety net	Food bank, food pantries, soup kitchens and food subsidies	• Location of food distribution outlets in "at risk" areas • Food distribution outlets have insufficient capacity, including storage, to meet demand • Food distribution outlets do not have contingency plans, including alternative supply chains and sufficient insurance • Sub-system outlet vulnerabilities (e.g., utilities) • Vulnerabilities associated with transporting consumers to food distribution outlets (e.g., infrastructure, public transportation) • Vulnerabilities associated with transporting food from food banks to distribution outlets (e.g., weak roads, vehicle supply) • Vulnerabilities associated with supply chains to food banks and food pantries • Insufficient or non-sustainable funding sources • Insufficient food subsidies for population or food basket prices • Food subsidy inflexibility (e.g., does not allow purchases for alternative products post-disaster) • Regulations

Processing and packaging

Concentrated ownership and location in "at risk" areas pose the greatest vulnerabilities for food processing. For example, if the processing of a food product is owned by a single company and that company goes out of business, it would obviously create supply issues. Food processing in the U.S. is increasingly concentrated (Ollinger et al. 2005). The 12 percent of food processing plants with more than 100 employees ship 77 percent of all of the value of food in the U.S. (Nesheim, Oria, and Yih 2015).

The location of food processing plants is also increasingly concentrated spatially, which means they are exposed to local natural disasters. For example, even with seasonal local production, lettuce production and packaging in the U.S. remains concentrated in California and Arizona, accounting for about 98 percent of commercial domestic output (Lucier and Jerardo 2006). Chicken production and processing is concentrated in the South (National Chicken Council 2015), often in integrated production complexes (MacDonald 2014). Fifty-three percent of chicken is produced by four firms: Tyson, Pilgrim's Pride, Sanderson Farms, and Perdue (Watt Poultry USA 2015), which together have approximately 95 chicken slaughterhouses and processing facilities in 18 states, the majority in Arkansas, Georgia and Texas (United States Department of Agriculture Food Safety and Inspection Service 2015).

In terms of non-perishable items, Campbell's Soup and Progresso, which is owned by General Mills, are the market leaders in canned condensed soup production. Campbell's Soup controls more than 60 percent of the market (Campbell Soup Company 2015), while Progresso controls 13.5 percent (Ellison 2013). Infant formula is another example of a concentrated market, with three major manufacturers (Mead Johnson, Nestle, and Abbott) controlling 98 percent of the market (Oliveira, Frazão, and Smallwood, 2011).

Transportation and distribution

Concentrated ownership and location also create vulnerabilities in urban food distribution, often compounded by outdated infrastructure for warehouses and markets. For example, in New York City, fresh food from across the world is brought into warehouses at the Hunts Point Distribution Center, a 329-acre facility in the Hunts Point Peninsula in the Bronx, before being distributed to grocery stores, corner stores, specialty shops and other retail outlets across the city. About 60 percent of the city's produce and about half of its meat and fish pass through Hunts Point. Built in 1967, Hunts Point's facilities and infrastructure are aging and outdated. For example, only about 50 percent of produce that goes through the Hunts Point Terminal Market is stored inside the warehouse facility; the remainder is stored in several hundred refrigerated diesel trucks on the property (Brannan 2010). Moreover, Hunts Point is surrounded by the East and Bronx Rivers on three sides, and is especially vulnerable to flooding and storm surges, with 28 percent of the Distribution Center located in a floodplain (PlaNYC 2013). While Hunts Point was not compromised during Superstorm Sandy in 2012, if the storm had taken a different path or arrived during high tide, the Center might have lost power and significant inventory, and suffered from major operational interruptions (PlaNYC 2013).

Nearly all food is distributed to retail points by truck, so the physical condition of roads, bridges and tunnels are critical points of vulnerability (Lawrence, Ritter, and Gergely 2011; The Road Information Program 2015). For example, any closure of the Golden Gate Bridge after an earthquake effectively disconnects the city of San Francisco from much of the Bay Area. Reliance on a single mode of transportation and a single pathway (i.e., trucks traveling on a single highway) also creates vulnerabilities. Superstorm Sandy closed several of New York's tunnels and bridges, including the critical George Washington Bridge over which 45 percent of deliveries to Hunts Point travel (URS and Goodkind and O'Dea n.d.). Overall, it is estimated that nearly 30 percent of truck traffic over that one bridge carries food (PlaNYC 2013).

Retail outlets

Depending on the city in question, most food purchases are at grocery stores, which are typically defined as offering a full-range of food items and are 7,000 square feet or larger, or at corner stores or bodegas, which are convenience stores or food marts that primarily offer a limited line of food items. However, food sales are increasing at drugstore chains such as CVS and retail chains such as Target. Among these various types of retail sources, corner stores and smaller grocery stores may face longer periods of closure after a natural disaster because they do not have access to national resources to help them tap into other supply chains. The majority of grocery stores are likely to have short-term contingency plans in place for a natural disaster, but may not be prepared for long-term or major supply chain disruptions. Corner stores are unlikely to have any contingency plans in place, and most would simply stay closed until supply chains returned to normal.

These disparate vulnerabilities will put some neighborhoods at greater risk depending on the type of stores serving them. In general, poorer neighborhoods have fewer large supermarkets and rely more on corner stores (Bower et al 2014; Treuhaft and Karpyn 2010). New Orleans, for example, has typically been served by local or regional grocery stores and few national chain grocery stores. The city lost half of its grocery stores after Katrina (from 31 in 2004 to 15 in 2007), a number that only returned to pre-Katrina levels in 2014, nearly ten years later (Thompson 2015). Most local and smaller grocery stores were not able to rebuild after Katrina because they did not have the capital or resources of a national chain to come back. For example, Circle Food Store, a local, independent grocery store in an underserved 7th Ward neighborhood, closed due to flooding damage. The owner did not have flood insurance and it took eight years for the store to reopen, with the help of new funds from the City designed to increase fresh food access in food deserts (Sayre 2014). In a few instances abandoned food retail spaces have been taken over by national chain stores such as Walmart and Whole Foods.

In some cities, such as New York, the diversity of grocery stores and corner stores (bodegas) creates some resilience. Having many and diverse grocery options was a factor in the continued functioning of food retail after Sandy. Only certain neighborhoods experienced disruption in food retail, and most residents were able to rely on additional grocery stores, sometimes a few miles away, for their food needs. On the other hand, smaller stores have limited storage capacity, and often deplete stock in a few days after a storm. Such stores also have limited access to supply chains, and may take longer to replenish their shelves (Mantanta 2013).

The distances consumers must travel to food retail outlets and food pantries create food access vulnerabilities. Although food may be available at stores and food pantries after a natural disaster, some consumers may not have reasonable access to them even in normal times. As such, food deserts in a normal state diminish food resilience because they limit food access. The U.S. Department of Agriculture (USDA) defines food deserts as census tracts with a substantial share of residents who live in low-income areas that have limited access to a grocery store or other healthy, affordable food retail outlets (Dutko, Ver Ploeg and Farrigan 2012). Within San Francisco, for example, 30,772 people (3.8 percent) live in a food desert, compared to only 9,947 people (0.1 percent) in New York City (U.S. Department of Agriculture 2013). Retail density and proximity matter to food access.

Food safety net

Other food systems vulnerabilities stem from the inability of consumers to afford food. Such residents tend to rely on food subsidies, such as the Supplemental Nutrition Assistance Program (SNAP) and the Special Supplemental Nutrition Program for Women, Infants, and Children (WIC) to purchase some food items, and many supplement their daily food needs from food pantries. Food banks and pantries already play a significant and increasing role as a safety net for food insecure households, and in the event of a natural disaster may not have the capacity or resources to meet increased demand over a longer time period. After Sandy, 60 percent of food pantries and soup kitchens in New York City reported that they were feeding more people at least partially due to Sandy one year after the storm. All agencies in Staten Island, one of the areas hardest hit by Sandy, reported feeding more people (New York City Coalition Against Hunter 2013).

Food banks belonging to Feeding America, a nationwide network of 200 member food banks and 60,000 food pantries, are able to access food from the national organization during disasters (Feeding America 2015). Feeding America plays an active role in recovery efforts following major disasters by providing local organizations with food, water and trained staff, while providing specialized disaster training for its food banks around the country. In 2005, Feeding America formalized its commitment to providing aid during times of disaster with the Federal Emergency Management Agency (FEMA) and played important roles during Hurricane Katrina and Superstorm Sandy. Feeding America provided more than 83 million pounds of supplies to the Gulf Coast in the months after Katrina. Local food pantries and meal programs, which rely on food banks, may not have similar contingency or disaster response plans.

Location in "at risk areas" is also a problem for food banks and meal programs. For example, the warehouse for Food Bank for New York City is located in Hunts

Point and is exposed to the area's flooding and infrastructure vulnerabilities. In addition, many of New York's food pantries and soup kitchens are located in church basements and experienced flooding during Sandy (PlaNYC 2013).

Lessons learned from Boston

We applied our framework to Boston during 2014–2015 (Initiative for a Competitive Inner City 2015). The resilience of Boston's food system to natural disasters is of increasing interest to the city in the wake of Superstorm Sandy, which narrowly missed Boston in 2012, and in the aftermath of the record-breaking snowfall in the early months of 2015.

Processing and packaging

Instead of asking where a city's food is grown, the more pertinent question to ask when analyzing the impact of a natural disaster is where is the city's food originating from at the point of processing and packaging? And who controls the supply chain? To find out, we chose a representative sample of five food items found in an average consumer grocery basket. It includes a relatively shelf-stable food item (bread), an item with a short shelf-life (milk), a fresh, leafy vegetable that is consumed fresh with a relatively short shelf-life and few opportunities for preservation (lettuce), an affordable protein (chicken), a packaged shelf-stable item (chicken noodle soup) and a specialized food item necessary for certain populations (infant formula).

Bread. Private label or store brands, in aggregate, account for 27 percent of all fresh bread sales in the U.S (Flowers Foods 2015). Anecdotal evidence from a food buyer suggests that the majority of commercial white bread sold in Boston is private label. Due to insufficient data, we were not able to determine the leading private label brands in Boson. Three brands, Bimbo Bakeries USA (a subsidiary of Grupo Bimbo of Mexico), Flowers Foods, and Pepperidge Farm are the primary national branded bread manufacturers, controlling over half of the fresh bread market (IRI 2015). Private label bread is often produced by leading bread manufacturers. For instance, Flowers Foods produces 15 percent of all private label bread sold in the United States (IRI 2015).

Milk. Most milk consumed in Boston is supplied and processed by two large dairy corporations. Dallas-based Suiza, which owns Dean Foods and Garelick Farms, supplies 63.7 percent of all grocery milk in New England and supplies nearly all of the private label milk in Boston (Cotterill and Franklin 2001: 44, 69). Boston-area based H.P. Hood supplies another 20.1 percent of all grocery milk in New England, including private label brands (Cotterill and Franklin 2001: 69).

Baby formula. Mead Johnson (Enfamil Infant) is the only WIC-approved provider of standard infant formula in Massachusetts, although the company's manufacturing plants are located in Michigan and Indiana. This monopoly creates vulnerabilities. As witnessed after Sandy, WIC regulations created difficulties with purchasing some food staples for New York City WIC recipients. After

Sandy, one distribution expert noted that there was a shortage of certain WIC-eligible food items, such as bread. WIC recipients were not able to purchase bread if it was the wrong size or type. In addition, in New York State, WIC recipients are required to buy all items listed on a WIC check. If the store did not have all items on the WIC check, a recipient could not use the benefit. Stores had to either sell these items to non-WIC customers or return food items to their suppliers for a credit, rather than selling to people receiving the benefit. This issue remained for two months after the storm.

Natural disasters, such as a hurricane or blizzard, will impact components of a city's food system outside of the City's limits, such as processing and packaging facilities and distribution. To assess locational vulnerabilities of these components in Boston, we looked at facilities in a 75-mile radius of the city, a range that roughly corresponds with the typical extent of hurricane force winds (National Weather Service National Hurricane Center 2015). However, the actual impacted area will vary by natural disaster type, path, magnitude and location.

Bread production tends to take place closer to customers. Bimbo Bakeries, which produces Arnold, Freihofer's and Sara Lee brands among others, has three locations in Massachusetts (IRI 2015). Flowers Foods, whose brands include Nature's Own, Sunbeam and Wonder, has five bakeries located in Maine, Vermont and Pennsylvania (Gelski 2014). However, most of Boston's supply of commercial white bread comes from beyond 75 miles. Only two major commercial bread bakeries and two private label/regional brand bakeries operate within a 75-mile radius of Boston.

Milk is perishable and has to be transported from farm to consumer relatively quickly. Like other cities, Boston's milk is supplied and processed by regional dairy farms and processing facilities; 9 percent of the milk processed in Massachusetts is supplied from Massachusetts dairy farms, 64 percent is from another New England state, and 27 percent is from outside of New England (Horwitz 2011). Overall, five state-certified raw or pasteurized fluid milk processing facilities in Massachusetts are located within 75 miles of Boston, as are another seven processing facilities permitted to ship milk into Massachusetts, including one in Connecticut, three in New Hampshire, and three in Rhode Island. Garelick Farms operates four major processing facilities in New England, two within 75 miles of Boston and the closest ten miles from Boston's city center (U.S. Food and Drug Administration 2015). In theory, Garelick would be well positioned to respond effectively if any one plant has to stop operations, but the record snowstorms in early 2015 surfaced potential vulnerabilities. In particular, with road traffic delayed by weather, federal Hours of Service (HOS) regulations significantly curtailed Garelick's overall distribution capacity. A company representative estimated that it took Garelick a full month to return to full capacity in terms of filling delivery orders to Boston following the initial major snowstorm, and that 20 percent of Boston's grocery stores were out of milk for at least 24 hours at some point during this event.

The supply of chicken, lettuce and infant formula is concentrated in the hands of few companies with more distant geographic locations, creating a different set of risks for Boston's food supply that should be addressed in future resilience planning efforts.

Distribution and transportation

Boston's food stores and institutions are supplied by a robust mix of integrated retail distribution systems, and by national, regional, and local distributors, with key distribution points spread across the region. As one industry expert explained, the city's large grocery stores, and national retailers that sell food, such as Target, rely on a mix of vertically integrated and third-party distribution centers for both fresh and shelf-stable food products. The city's local fresh food distributors cater to both large grocery stores and corner stores in different capacities. The larger stores may rely on local fresh food distributors directly or indirectly for certain products or at certain times of the year. The city's corner stores rely on a mix of third-party distribution centers or direct access (i.e., buying product directly from local or regional distributors).

Local fresh food distributors have smaller, specialized warehouses that are clustered in several locations in and around Boston. For example, the distributors located in Chelsea and Everett, inner urban suburbs neighboring Boston, predominantly sell produce. The New England Produce Center (in Chelsea) was built in 1968 and contains 128 store units. It is the largest privately held produce market in the country. Literally next door to it, in Everett, is the Boston Market Terminal. The two markets are near capacity serving a growing population (Nelson 2012). Distributors located in the south Boston Newmarket area primarily sell meat and seafood, although some also sell produce and baked goods. The Port of Boston plays an important role in importing some food commodities by boat (e.g., frozen fish), which are then distributed locally via truck (Massachusetts Department of Transportation 2010: 2–105).

While the relatively decentralized nature of food distribution in Boston limits some risks associated with natural disasters, their location in or near floodplains creates others. The New England Produce Center is located in a FEMA designated "low- to moderate-risk" flood zone. Overall, 45 percent of the fresh food wholesalers serving Boston would likely flood if a 7.5-foot storm surge hit Boston during high tide.[2]

The majority of Boston's food (94 percent) arrives by truck. As is typical in many older U.S. cities, many of Boston's main roadways are at capacity and deteriorating. Congestion impacts for both passenger and freight vehicles are projected to increase significantly in the metropolitan Boston region and statewide. Forty-nine percent of Boston area roads are rated as in substandard condition (Massachusetts Department of Transportation 2010). There are only two state and federal designated truck routes in Boston, I-90 and I-93. In Boston, nearly all of I-93, the critical North–South route that includes the Central Artery tunnel system in downtown Boston, is projected to be vulnerable to coastal flooding via coastal storms and sea level rise (Spector and Bamberger 2013: 21). One industry expert noted that because most distribution points are located outside of Boston, I-93 is the primary transportation route for food into the city.

Boston's old and narrow secondary streets pose another source of risk in the food distribution system. The feeder roads to some distributors were not designed to handle the traffic volume and are deteriorating, creating traffic congestion issues (Nelson 2012). Streets that were further narrowed due to snow build-up during the 2015 winter storms also made it difficult for trucks to pass, causing delivery delays.

Retail outlets

Boston's food retail outlets comprise a mix of large national, regional, and local grocery stores as well as many corner stores. At the time of this analysis there were 40 grocery stores, with at least four more in development, and 240 corner stores in Boston (Lima et al. 2013; City of Boston 2013). The grocery stores are owned by 16 unique companies, although 53 percent are owned by three large chains (Lima et al. 2013).

Unique for large cities, most residential neighborhoods in Boston have at least one grocery store, and 99 percent of Boston residents live within a half mile of a corner store.[3] Over 70 percent of residents live within one mile of more than one grocery store option.[4] Residents are also well served by corner stores. On average, there are 1.6 grocery stores per neighborhood and 0.06 grocery stores per capita in Boston.[5] There are 9.6 corner stores per neighborhood on average and there are 0.39 corner stores per capita in Boston.[6] As a result, only two census tracts within Boston city limits, containing 9,196 people (1.5 percent), officially qualify as food deserts (U.S. Department of Agriculture 2015).

Most of Boston's food retail outlets are located in areas that are not at risk of flooding; no grocery stores are located in a FEMA floodplain or five-foot storm surge zone. Twenty-three percent of the grocery stores, however, could flood if a 7.5-foot storm surge hit during high tide. Only two corner stores are located in the FEMA floodplain – but nearly a quarter of the corner stores, in 13 neighborhoods, could flood if a 7.5 foot storm surge hit during high tide.

Although the decentralized, robust food retail and distribution network in Boston makes its food system comparatively resilient, it poses challenges for planning and coordination. A number of organizations and associations exist that represent the food retail and distribution network, and their coordination with each other and with City agencies remains informal. The Massachusetts Food Association, a nonprofit trade association for the state's supermarket and grocery industry, has membership that includes large chain supermarkets and wholesalers in and near Boston; however, their members do not include some of the city's independent grocery stores. The Latin American Grocers Association represents some of the smaller corner stores. The Newmarket Business Association represents the wholesalers, as well as other businesses, in the Newmarket area. While these associations interact with the City in various capacities, no known formal resilience coordination is in place. For example, the Massachusetts Food

Association (MFA) is well connected with the state government, and coordinates with the Massachusetts Emergency Management Agency during disasters; however, no coordination takes place between the MFA and the City of Boston's Office of Emergency Management, nor with city agencies responsible for resilience or climate change planning.

One potential issue that stronger public-private coordination could solve is an increase in demand from neighborhood stores due to a natural disaster. For example, a long-term closure of public schools after a disaster would likely increase demand for food from retail outlets. There are 128 K-12 public schools in Boston that serve breakfast and lunch to 57,000 students (Boston Public Schools 2015b). Seventy-eight percent of BPS students qualify for free or reduced lunch and breakfast (Boston Public Schools 2015a). One school is located in a FEMA floodplain, while 28 more would likely flood if a 7.5-foot storm surge hit Boston during high tide (Spector and Bamberger 2013). One year after Katrina, only one-third of New Orleans public schools had reopened (Liu, Fellowes, and Mabanta 2006), and many did not reopen at all.

Food security safety net

Food access varies significantly across Boston's neighborhoods. Just over 18 percent of the city's population is living at or below poverty level and just over 18 percent of households receive SNAP benefits (U.S. Census Bureau 2013).[7] Eight neighborhoods have poverty rates higher than the city average. Six neighborhoods have household SNAP participation rates higher than the average.[8] An estimated 15.8 percent of individuals in Suffolk County (where Boston is located) are rated as food insecure, the highest rate in Massachusetts (Gundersen et al. 2015). A natural disaster may also push more people into SNAP eligibility income thresholds, long-term, due to potential decreases in income (e.g., job loss).

Many food insecure individuals rely on food pantries and other feeding organizations for a portion of their food needs. There are 79 food pantries in Boston that are members of The Greater Boston Food Bank (GBFB), 58 percent of which are located in three inner city neighborhoods. The Food Bank is housed in a state-of-the-art, 117,000-square-foot distribution center built in 2009 (The Greater Boston Food Bank 2015a). It has over 500 member agencies that serve 500,000 people annually across Eastern Massachusetts (The Greater Boston Food Bank 2014). Food is delivered daily to and from GBFB. A representative from GBFB estimates that approximately 75 percent of its members pick up food weekly at GBFB. The remainder is delivered by GBFB. The representative noted that currently GBFB does not have sufficient capacity or storage to meet demand and will sometimes need to use offsite freezer facilities. In 2014, The Greater Boston Food Bank distributed 50 million pounds of food, putting the new facility at full capacity well before it was estimated to reach that mark (The Greater Boston Food Bank 2011). The Greater Boston Food Bank has also seen an increase in demand for produce, creating storage issues. When the new GBFB facility was built, only 2 percent of food was expected to be produce. Today, produce accounts for 25 percent of GBFB's food.

The unique role The Greater Boston Food Bank plays in supporting the broad food safety network in Boston poses its own set of vulnerabilities. If it is closed or has limited access, food pantries will have less food. Ninety-one percent of GBFB member agencies said a decrease in food received from The Greater Boston Food Bank would negatively impact their ability to serve clients (The Greater Boston Food Bank 2015b). The reliance of many organizations on a single source for most of its food needs creates risks of supply disruptions.

The physical location of The Greater Boston Food Bank also presents significant transportation issues. Wedged in the Newmarket section of the city, GBFB has to work with other Newmarket business owners to coordinate the use of private access roads by food delivery trucks. The 2015 winter storms revealed some additional vulnerabilities; snow buildup on the narrow feeder roads made it difficult for food delivery trucks and member agencies to get to GBFB.

The Greater Boston Food Bank is central to any food system resilience planning. It has a Vice President of Food Acquisition and Supply Chain with previous private supply chain management experience for a major grocery store to oversee its food acquisitions. The position works with grocers and suppliers to both purchase food and secure large food donations. Its relationship with the private sector positions GBFB to coordinate with grocery stores during disasters. It also coordinates with the Massachusetts Emergency Management Agency and is a member of the Massachusetts Voluntary Organizations Active in Disaster, a forum where organizations share knowledge and resources before, throughout, and after a disaster (Massachusetts Voluntary Organizations Active in Disaster 2015). Finally, the Greater Boston Food Bank has a formal disaster response plan in place, which outlines the steps needed to ensure continuity of services and how it will serve the community.

Final thoughts

While American cities are beginning to pay more attention to natural disaster vulnerabilities, they are focused on obvious factors (e.g., infrastructure) and overlook a critical component – food systems. Our research in Boston, coupled with the impact of the natural disasters in New York City and New Orleans, highlight crucial vulnerabilities in urban food systems that could cause significant food supply disruptions. City leaders clearly need to prioritize food resilience and yet they lack the data and capacity to undertake a thorough analysis of their entire food system. The challenge is compounded by the fact that most of the food system is comprised of private companies and proprietary information. The framework and approach described above can help cities identify areas of vulnerability to prioritize for more in-depth study.

As the Boston research highlights, city leaders concerned about climate change need to consider vulnerabilities along the entire food supply chain, especially processing and distribution, and not just focus on substituting imported food with local production. Food access and insecurity issues affect food resilience in important ways and underscore the need to understand vulnerabilities at the neighborhood level. As we learned from Katrina, the most vulnerable populations in cities will be disproportionately impacted by natural disasters. The same will be true for Boston. As urban populations continue to grow, they will put more stress on food distribution systems, making them inherently less resilient to severe storm events. City leaders need to incorporate food systems into their resilience planning, but public-private cooperation will be required to address this issue and make urban food systems more resilient.

Notes

1   100 Resilient Cities. 2016. "Selected Cities." Available online at www.100resilientcities. org/cities (accessed March 4, 2016).
2   Federal Emergency Management Agency, "National Flood Hazard Layer," MassGIS, last modified 2014; Initiative for a Competitive Inner City, Next Street, and Karp Resources, "Designing an Inner City Food Cluster Strategy" (2012); Paul Kirshen, Ellen Douglas, and Chris Watson, "Boston Harbor Sea Level Rise Maps" (The Boston Harbor Association, 2013); ICIC Analysis.
3   "Corner Stores," City of Boston Mayor's Office of Food Initiatives, Data Boston, last modified January 30, 2013. Available online at https://data.cityofboston.gov/dataset/ Corner-Stores/4vcu-nshu (accessed September 7, 2016); U.S. Census Bureau 2013 American Community Survey 5-Year Estimates; ICIC Analysis.
4   Lima, et al. 2013; U.S. Census Bureau, 2013 American Community Survey 5-Year Estimates; ICIC Analysis.
5   "Boston Neighborhood Shapefiles," Boston Redevelopment Authority, Data Boston, last modified January 24, 2014. Available online at https://data.cityofboston.gov/City-Services/Boston-Neighborhood-Shapefiles/af56-j7tb (accessed September 7, 2016); Boston Redevelopment Authority Research Division, *Neighborhood Profiles: City of Boston* (Boston Redevelopment Authority, 2014); Alvaro Lima, Mark Melnik, Kelly Dowd, and Joanne Wong, *Grocery Stores in Boston* (Boston: Boston Redevelopment Authority, 2013); ICIC Analysis.
6   "Boston Neighborhood Shapefiles," Boston Redevelopment Authority, Data Boston, last modified January 24, 2014. Available online at https://data.cityofboston.gov/City-Services/Boston-Neighborhood-Shapefiles/af56-j7tb (accessed September 7, 2016); Boston Redevelopment Authority Research Division, Neighborhood Profiles: City of Boston (Boston: Boston Redevelopment Authority, 2014); "Corner Stores," City of Boston Mayor's Office of Food Initiatives, Data Boston, last modified January 30, 2013. Available online at https://data.cityofboston.gov/dataset/Corner-Stores/4vcu-nshu (accessed September 7, 2016); ICIC Analysis.
7   Poverty rate estimates exclude currently enrolled undergraduate and graduate students. We exclude Boston's substantial college population because it skews poverty rate estimates, and students are likely to leave the city in the event of a disaster-related school closure.
8   Boston Redevelopment Authority, "2010 Census Tracts & Neighborhoods" (Boston Redevelopment Authority, 2014); U.S. Census Bureau 2013 American Community Survey 5-Year Estimates; ICIC Analysis.

References

Bennet, C. 2012. "Food Trucks Rolling." *Metro*, October 31. Available online at http://nypost.com/2012/10/31/food-trucks-rolling/ (accessed September 7, 2016).

Boston Public Schools. 2015a. "BPS Offers Universal Free Meals for Every Child." Available online at www.bostonpublicschools.org/domain/238 (accessed April 14, 2016).

Boston Public Schools. 2015b. "Facts, Figures and Reports." Available online at http://www.bostonpublicschools.org/domain/238 (accessed July 11, 2016).

Bower, K., Thorpe R., Rohde, C., and Gaskin D. 2014. "The intersection of neighborhood racial segregation, poverty and urbanicity, and its impact on food store availability in the United States." *Preventative Medicine* 58 (1): 33–39.

Brannan, S. 2010. *Food Works: A Vision to Improve NYC's Food System*. New York, NY: The New York City Council.

Bristow, D. and Kennedy, C. 2013. "Urban metabolism and the energy stored in cities: Implications for resilience." *Journal of Industrial Ecology* 17 (5): 656–667.

Campbell Soup Company. 2015. "About Us." Available online at http://www.campbellsoup.com/Resources/AboutUs (accessed April 15, 2016).

City of Boston, Mayor's Office of Food Initiatives. 2013. "Corner Stores." Available online at https://data.cityofboston.gov/dataset/Corner-Stores/4vcu-nshu (accessed July 11, 2016).

Cotterill, R. and Frankin, A. 2001. *The Public Interest and Private Economic Power: A Case Study of the Northeast Dairy Compact*. Storrs, CT: Food Marketing Policy Center, Department of Agricultural and Resource Economics, University of Connecticut.

Dutko, P., Ver Ploeg, M., and Farrigan, T. 2012. *Characteristics and Influential Factors of Food Deserts, ERR-140*. Washington, DC: U.S. Department of Agriculture, Economic Research Service.

Ellison, S. 2013. "Campbell's Big Bet: Heating up Condensed Soup, Battling Progresso." *The Wall Street Journal*, July 31. Available online at www.wsj.com/articles/SB105959895913831100 (accessed April 12, 2015).

Fan, S., Pandya-Lorch, R. and Yosef, R. (eds.) 2014. *Resilience for Food and Nutrition Security*. Washington, DC: International Food Policy Research Institute.

Federal Emergency Management Agency. 2009. "FEMA Administrator Renews Partnership with Feeding America." October 22. Available online at www.fema.gov/news-release/2009/10/22/fema-administrator-renews-partnership-feeding-america (accessed March 4, 2016).

Feeding America. 2012. "Feeding America Prepares for Hurricane Sandy." Last modified October 29. Available online at www.feedingamerica.org/hunger-in-america/news-and-updates/press room/press-releases/feeding-america-prepares-for-hurricane-sandy.html (accessed April 12, 2015).

Feeding America. 2015. "Food Bank Network." Available online at www.feedingamerica.org/our-response/how-we-work/food-bank-network/ (accessed April 11, 2016).

Flowers Food. 2015. *Flowers Foods Investor Fact Sheet*: February 2015. Thomasville, GA.

Food Bank NYC. 2015. "About Food Bank." Available online at www.foodbanknyc.org/about-food-bank (accessed April 14, 2016).

Gelski, J. 2014. "Flowers Names Senior V.P. for Northeast Region." *Baking Business*, July 22. Available online at www.bakingbusiness.com/articles/news_home/People/2014/07/Flowers_names_snior_vp_for_No.aspx?ID=%7BD9D99503-87E1-4309-9172-24C11CF553F5%7D (accessed September 7, 2016).

Green, J. (ed.) 2012. Special Issue: Community Responses to Disaster. *Community Development* 43 (5), 540–549.

Gundersen, C., Satoh, A., Dewey, A., Kato, M., and Engelhard, E. 2015. *Map the Meal Gap 2015: Overall Food Insecurity in Massachusetts by County in 2013*. Chicago, IL: Feeding America.

The Greater Boston Food Bank. 2011. "The Greater Boston Food Bank Completes $35 Million Fighting Hunger, Feeding Hope Capital Campaign." Press Release, February 11.

The Greater Boston Food Bank. 2014. *Hunger in Eastern Massachusetts 2014*. Boston, MA.

The Greater Boston Food Bank. 2015a. "About GBFB." Available online at www.gbfb. org/our-mission/about-gbfb.php (accessed April 14, 2016).

The Greater Boston Food Bank. 2015b. "Hunger Study." Available online at www.gbfb. org/our-mission/hunger.php (accessed April 12, 2016).

The Greater Boston Food Bank, Inc. and Subsidiary. 2014. *Consolidated Financial Statements (With Supplementary Information) and Independent Auditor's Report*. Boston, MA.

Hatfield, J., Takle, G., Grotjahn, R., Holden, P., Cesar Izaurralde, R., Mader, T., Marshall, E., and Liverman, D. 2014. "Agriculture," in *Climate Change Impacts in the United States: The Third National Climate Assessment*, edited by J.M. Melillo, T. Richmond, and G.W. Yohe, 150–174; U.S. Global Change Research Program.

Horwitz, R. 2011. "Massachusetts Workshop on FMD Vulnerability and Preparedness." Presentation.

Initiative for a Competitive Inner City. 2015. Resilient Food Systems, Resilient Cities: Recommendations for the City of Boston. Boston, MA.

IRI. 2015. *Flowers Food Investor Fact Sheet*. Flowers Foods.

Lawrence, T., Ritter, C., and Gergely, J. 2011. "Bridge Monitoring and Performance Evaluation." *Geotechnical and Geological Engineering* 29: 919–926.

Lima, A., Melnik, M., Dowd, K., and Wong, J. 2013. *Grocery Stores in Boston*. Boston: Boston Redevelopment Authority.

Liu, A., Fellowes, M. and Mabanta, M. 2006. *Special Edition of the Katrina Index: A One-Year Review of Key Indicators of Recovery in Post-Storm New Orleans*. Washington DC: The Brookings Institution.

Lucier, G. and Jerardo, A. 2006. *Vegetables and Melons Outlook VGS-315*. Washington, DC: U.S. Department of Agriculture, Economic Research Service.

MacDonald, J. 2014. *Technology, Organization, and Financial Performance in U.S. Broiler Production*. Report no. EIB-126. United States Department of Agriculture, Economic Research Service.

Mahanta, S. 2013. "A year after Sandy, food and fuel supplies are as vulnerable as ever." *Reuters*, October 28. Available online at http://blogs.reuters.com/great-debate/2013/10/28/a-year-after-sandy-food-and-fuel-supplies-as-vulnerable-as-ever/ (accessed May 25, 2016).

Malcolm, S., Marshall, E., Aillery, M., Heisey, P., Livingston, M., and Day-Rubenstein, K. 2012. *Agricultural Adaptation to a Changing Climate: Economic and Environmental Implications Vary by U.S. Region, ERR-136*. Washington, DC: U.S. Department of Agriculture, Economic Research Service.

Mantanta, S. 2013. "New York's Looming Food Disaster." *Citylab*, October 21. Available online at www.citylab.com/politics/2013/10/new-yorks-looming-food-disaster/7294/ (accessed May 25, 2016).

Massachusetts Department of Transportation. 2010. *Massachusetts Department of Transportation Freight Plan*. Boston, MA.

Massachusetts Executive Office Energy and Environmental Affairs. 2015. "Massachusetts Emergency Food Assistance Program." Available online at www.mass.gov/eea/agencies/agr/about/divisions/mefap.html (accessed April 13, 2016).

Massachusetts Voluntary Organizations Active in Disaster. 2015. "About VOAD." Available online at http://massvoad.org/news/?page_id=55. (accessed April 13, 2016).

National Chicken Council. 2015. "Top Broiler Producing States." Available online at www.nationalchickencouncil.org/about-the-industry/statistics/top-broiler-producing-states/ (accessed April 14, 2016).

National Weather Service National Hurricane Center. 2015. "Strike." *Glossary of NHC Terms*. Available online at www.nhc.noaa.gov/aboutgloss.shtml (accessed April 11, 2016).

Nelson, A. 2012. "Wholesalers Happy with Terminal Markets." *The Packer*, March 22. Available online at www.thepacker.com/fruit-vegetable-news/know-your-market/Wholesalers-happy-with-terminal-markets-143833566.html (accessed April 11, 2016).

Nesheim, M., Oria, M., and Tsai Yih, P. 2015. "Overview of the U.S. Food System," in *A Framework for Assessing Effects of the Food System*. Washington, DC: The National Academies Press.

New York City Coalition Against Hunger. 2013. Superstorm of Hunger. New York, NY.

Oliveira, V., Frazão, E., and Smallwood, D. 2011. *The Infant Formula Market: Consequences of a Change in the WIC Contract Brand, ERR-124*. Washington, DC: U.S. Department of Agriculture, Economic Research Service.

Ollinger, M., Nguyen, S. V., Blayney, D., Chambers, B., and Nelson, K. 2005. *Structural Change in the Meat, Poultry, Dairy and Grain Processing Industries*. Washington, DC: U.S. Department of Agriculture, Economic Research Service.

Otto, A., Schoppengerd, F., and Shariatmadari, R. 2009. "Success in the Consumer Products Market: Understanding Direct Store Delivery," in *Direct Store Delivery: Concepts, Applications and Instruments*, edited by A. Otto, F.J. Schoppengerd, and R. Shariatmadari. Berlin: Springer-Verlag, 1–30.

PlaNYC. 2013. *A Stronger, More Resilient New York*. New York, NY.

The Road Information Program. 2015. *Bumpy Roads Ahead: America's Roughest Rides and Strategies to Make Our Roads Smoother*. Washington, DC: Transportation Research Board of the National Academies.

San Francisco Food Security Task Force. 2013. *Assessment of Food Security in San Francisco*. San Francisco, CA.

Sayre, K. 2014. "Circle Food Store opens again after eight-year struggle to rebuild." *The Times-Picayune*. January 17, 2014. Available online at www.nola.com/business/index.ssf/2014/01/circle_food_store_opens_again.html (accessed May 25, 2016).

Spector, C., and Bamberger, L. 2013. *Climate Ready Boston*. Boston, MA: Greenovate Boston.

Thompson, R. 2015. "Makin' groceries: Number of stores in New Orleans returns to pre-Katrina levels." *The Advocate*. August 13. Available online at http://theadvocate.com/news/neworleans/13171433-148/number-of-grocery-stores-in (accessed March 3, 2016).

Treuhaft, S, and Karpyn, A. 2010. *The Grocery Gap: Who Has Access to Healthy Food and Why It Matters*. Oakland, CA: PolcyLink.

Tyler, S., Keller, M., Swanson, D., Bizikova, L., Hammill, A., Zamudio, A. N., Moench, M., Dixit, A., Guevara Flores, R., Heer, C., González, D., Rivera Sosa, A., Murillo Gough, A., Solórzano, J. L., Wilson, C., Hernandez, X., and Bushey, S. 2013. *Climate Resilience and Food Security: A Framework for Planning and Monitoring*. Winnepeg, Canada: The International Institute for Sustainable Development.

United States Bureau of the Census. 2013. American Community Survey 5-Year Estimates; ICIC Analysis.

United States Food and Drug Administration. 2015. *IMS List: Sanitation and Compliance Enforcement Ratings of Interstate Milk Shippers January 2015*; ICIC Analysis.

United States Department of State. 2014. *United States Climate Action Report 2014.*

United States Department of Agriculture. 2013. "Food Access Research Atlas." Available online at www.ers.usda.gov/data-products/food-access-research-atlas/go-to-the-atlas. aspx (accessed April 13, 2015).

United States Department of Agriculture, Food Safety and Inspection Service. 2015. "Meat, Poultry and Egg Product Inspection Directory." Available online at www.fsis. usda.gov/wps/portal/fsis/topics/inspection/mpi-directory (accessed April 10, 2016).

URS and Goodkind & O'Dea, Inc. n.d. *Hunts Point Truck Study.* New York, NY.

Walthall, C. L., Hatfield, J., Backlund, P., Lengnick, L., Marshall, E., Walsh, M., Adkins, S., Aillery, M., Ainsworth, E. A., Ammann, C., Anderson, C. J., Bartomeus, I., Baumgard, L. H., Booker, F., Bradley, B., Blumenthal, D. M., Bunce, J., Burkey, K., Dabney, S. M., Delgado, J. A., Dukes, J., Funk, A., Garrett, K., Glenn, M., Grantz, D. A., Goodrich, D., Hu, S., Izaurralde, R. C., Jones, R. A. C., Kim, S-H., Leaky, A. D. B., Lewers, K., Mader, T. L., McClung, A., Morgan, J., Muth, D. J., Nearing, M., Oosterhuis, D. M., Ort, D., Parmesan, C., Pettigrew, W. T., Polley, W., Rader, R., Rice, C., Rivington, M., Rosskopf, E., Salas, W.A., Sollenberger, L. E., Srygley, R., Stöckle, C., Takle, E.S., Timlin, D., White, J. W., Winfree, R., Wright-Morton, L., and Ziska, L. H. 2012. *Climate Change and Agriculture in the United States: Effects and Adaptation.* Washington, DC: U.S. Department of Agriculture, Agriculture Research Service.

Watt Poultry USA. 2015. "USA's Top Broiler Companies." Available online at www. wattagnet.com/Marketdata/topcompanies/uspoultry/ (accessed April 15, 2016).

Weir, M., Pindus, N., Wial, H., and Wolman, H. (eds.) 2012. *Urban and Regional Policy and its Effects*: *Building Resilient Regions*, vol. 4. Washington, DC: The Brookings Institution.

Index

Page numbers in **bold** refer to figures, page numbers in *italic* refer to tables.

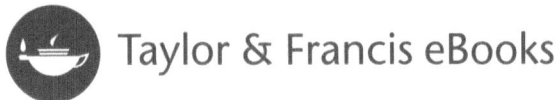
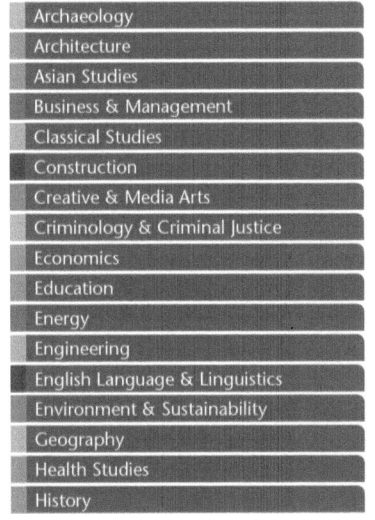
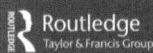